HIGH FIBER HIGH PROTEIN LOW CALORIE COOKBOOK

Gain Control of Your Digestive Health,
Lose Weight Quickly, Build Muscles,
and Live Long

CAROLINE SIMMONS, MD

Copyright Page

Copyright © 2024 by Caroline Simmons, MD.

All rights reserved. No part of this book may be reproduced, stored in a retrieval system, or transmitted in any form or by any means, electronic, mechanical, photocopying, recording, or otherwise, without the prior written permission of the author, except in the case of brief quotations embodied in critical articles and reviews.

The recipes and suggestions provided in this book are for informational purposes only. The author and publisher are not responsible for any adverse effects or consequences resulting from the use of the recipes, dietary practices, or suggestions described herein. Always consult a professional or medical expert if you have any concerns regarding your dietary needs and health conditions.

Table of Contents

1

MACRONUTRIENTS AND THEIR ROLE IN WEIGHT MANAGEMENT

Nutrients are substances required by the body to perform its basic functions. Most nutrients must be obtained from our diet, since the human body does not synthesize or produce them. Nutrients have one or more of three basic functions: they provide energy, contribute to body structure, and/or regulate chemical processes in the body. These basic functions allow us to detect and respond to environmental surroundings, move, excrete wastes, respire (breathe), grow, and reproduce.

There are six classes of nutrients required for the body to function and maintain overall health. These are: carbohydrates, lipids, proteins, water, vitamins, and minerals. Nutritious foods provide nutrients for the body. Foods may also contain a variety of non-nutrients. Some non-nutrients such as as antioxidants (found in many plant foods) are beneficial to the body, whereas others such as natural toxins (common in some plant foods) or additives (like certain dyes and preservatives found in processed foods) are potentially harmful.

What are Macronutrients?

Nutrients that are needed in large amounts are called macronutrients. There are three classes of macronutrients: carbohydrates, lipids, and proteins. Macronutrients are carbon-based compounds that can be metabolically processed into cellular energy through changes in their chemical bonds. The chemical energy is converted into cellular energy known as ATP (*Adenosine triphosphate*) that is utilized by the body to perform work and conduct basic functions.

The amount of energy a person consumes daily comes primarily from the 3 macronutrients. Food energy is measured in kilocalories. For ease of use, food labels state the amount of energy in food in "calories," meaning that each calorie is actually multiplied by one thousand to equal a kilocalorie. (Note: Using scientific terminology, "Calorie" (with a capital "C") is equivalent to a kilocalorie. Therefore: 1 kilocalorie = 1 Calorie - 1000 calories

Water is also a macronutrient in the sense that the body needs it in large amounts, but unlike the other macronutrients, it does not contain carbon or yield energy.

The Macronutrients: Carbohydrates, Lipids, Protein, and Water.

Carbohydrates

Carbohydrates are molecules composed of carbon, hydrogen, and oxygen that provide energy to the body. The major food sources of carbohydrates are milk, grains, fruits, and starchy vegetables, like potatoes. Non-starchy vegetables also contain carbohydrates, but in lesser quantities. Carbohydrates are broadly classified into two forms based on their chemical structure: simple carbohydrates (often called simple sugars) and complex carbohydrates.

Simple carbohydrates consist of one or two basic sugar units linked together. Their scientific names are "monosaccharides" (1 sugar unit) and disaccharides (2 sugar units). They are broken down and absorbed very quickly in the digestive tract and provide a fast burst of energy to the body. Examples of simple sugars include the disaccharide sucrose, the type of sugar you would have in a bowl on the breakfast table, and the monosaccharide glucose, the most common type of fuel for most organisms including humans. Glucose is the primary sugar that circulates in blood to provide energy to cells. The terms "blood sugar" and "blood glucose" can be substituted for each other.

Complex carbohydrates are long chains of sugars units that can link in a straight chair or a branched chain. During digestion, the body breaks down digestible complex carbohydrates into simple sugars, mostly glucose. Glucose is then absorbed into the bloodstream and transported to all our cells where it is stored, used to make energy, or used to build macromolecules. Fiber is also a complex carbohydrate, but it cannot be broken down by digestive enzymes in the human intestine. As a result, it passes through the digestive tract undigested unless the bacteria that inhabit the colon or large intestine break it down.

One gram of digestible carbohydrates yields 4 kilocalories of energy for the cells in the body to perform work. In addition to providing energy and serving as building blocks for bigger macromolecules, carbohydrates are essential for proper functioning of the nervous system, heart, and kidneys. As mentioned, glucose can be stored in the body for future use. In humans, the storage molecule of carbohydrates is called glycogen, and in plants, it is known as starch. Glycogen and starch are complex carbohydrates.

Lipids

Lipids are also a family of molecules composed of carbon, hydrogen, and oxygen, but unlike carbohydrates, they are insoluble in water. Lipids are found predominantly in butter, oils, meats, dairy products, nuts, and seeds, and in many processed foods. The three main types of lipids are triglycerides (triacylglycerols), phospholipids, and sterols. The main job of triacylglycerols is to provide or store energy. Lipids provide more energy per gram than carbohydrates (9 kilocalories per gram of lipids versus 4 kilocalories per gram of carbohydrates). In addition to energy storage, lipids serve as a major component of cell membranes, surround and protect organs (in fat-storing tissues), provide insulation to aid in temperature regulation. Phospholipds and sterols have a somewhat different chemical structure and are used to regulate many other functions in the body.

Proteins

Proteins are macromolecules composed of chains of basic subunits called amino acids. Amino acids are composed of carbon, oxygen, hydrogen, and nitrogen. Food sources of proteins include meats, dairy products, seafood, and a variety of different plant-based foods, most notably soy. The word protein comes from a Greek word meaning "of primary importance," which is an apt description of these macronutrients; they are also known colloquially as the "workhorses" of life. Proteins provide the basic structure to bones, muscles and skin, enzymes and hormones and play a role in conducting most of the chemical reactions that take place in the body. Scientists estimate that greater than one-hundred thousand different proteins exist within the human body. The genetic codes in DNA are basically protein recipes that determine the order in which 20 different amino acids are bound together to make thousands of specific proteins. Because amino acids contain carbon, they can be used by the body for energy and supply 4 kilocalories of energy per gram; however providing energy is not protein's most important function.

Water

There is one other nutrient that we must have in large quantities: water. Water does not contain carbon, but is composed of two hydrogen atoms and one oxygen atom per molecule of water. More than 60 percent of your total body weight is water. Without water, nothing could be transported in or out of the body, chemical reactions would not occur, organs would not be cushioned, and body temperature would widely fluctuate. On average, an adult consumes just over two liters of water per day from both eating foods and drinking liquids. Since water is so critical for life's basic processes, total water intake and output is supremely important.

Importance of macronutrients

Each type of macronutrient performs an important role in keeping the body healthy. For optimum health, people typically require a balance of macronutrients.

Macronutrient functions

Each macronutrient has specific functions in your body.

During digestion, they're broken down into smaller parts. These parts are then used for bodily functions like energy production, muscle building, and giving structure to cells.

Carbohydrates (Carbs)

Most carbs are broken down into glucose, or sugar molecules. This doesn't apply to dietary fiber, a type of carbohydrate that isn't broken down and passes through your body undigested. Still, some fiber is fermented by bacteria in your colon

Some of the main functions of carbs include:

Instant energy: Glucose is the preferred energy source for your brain, central nervous system, and red blood cells.

Storing energy: Glucose is stored as glycogen in your muscles and liver for later use when you need energy, for example after a longer period of fasting.

Digestion: Fiber promotes healthy bowel movements.

Helps you feel full: Fiber fills you up after eating and keeps you feeling full for longer.

Proteins

Proteins are digested into amino acids. Twenty amino acids have important functions in your body, 9 of which are essential and must be obtained from foods.

Some of the main uses of amino acids from protein include:

Building and repairing: Amino acids help create new proteins within your body. They're also used to build and repair tissues and muscles.

Providing structure: Amino acids provide structure to your body's cell membranes, organs, hair, skin, and nails.

pH balance: Amino acids help maintain a proper acid-base balance within your body.

Creating enzymes and hormones: Without the right amino acids, your body cannot create enzymes and hormones.

Fats (Lipids)

Fats are broken down into fatty acids and glycerol.

Some of the main functions of lipids, or fats, include:

Cell membrane health: Lipids are an essential component of cell membranes.

Storing energy: Fat stored around your body serves as an energy reserve that can be used during periods during which you eat fewer calories than you burn.

Transport and absorption: Lipids help transport and promote the absorption of the fat-soluble vitamins K, E, D, and A.

Insulation: Fat insulates and protects your organs.

Food sources of Carbs, Protein, and Fat

You can obtain macronutrients from the foods you eat. It's important to eat a variety of foods to get enough of each macronutrient.

Most foods contain a combination of carbs, protein, and fat.

Some foods are high in one specific macronutrient, while other foods contain high amounts of two nutrients and fall into two macronutrient groups.

Sources of carbs include:

Whole grains: brown rice, oats, farro, and barley

Vegetables: peas, potatoes, corn, and other starchy veggies

Fruits: mangoes, bananas, figs, and apples

Beans and legumes: black beans, lentils, and chickpeas

Dairy products: milk and yogurt

Sources of protein include:

Poultry: chicken and turkey

Eggs: particularly egg whites

Red meat: beef, lamb, and pork

Seafood: salmon, shrimp, and cod

Dairy products: milk, yogurt, and cheese

Beans and legumes: black beans, lentils, and chickpeas

Nuts and seeds: almonds and pumpkin seeds

Soy products: tofu, edamame, and tempeh

Sources of fat include:

Extra virgin olive oil

Coconut: fresh, dried, and coconut oil

Avocados: fresh and avocado oil

Nuts and seeds: almonds and pumpkin seeds

Fatty fish: salmon and herring

Dairy products: full fat yogurt and cheese

How to balance macronutrients for optimal weight management

How much to consume

Each macronutrient is incredibly important for your body to function optimally. It's crucial that you get enough carbs, protein, and fat by eating a balanced diet comprising a variety of foods.

Specifically, the United States Department of Agriculture (USDA) Dietary Guidelines recommend these Acceptable Macronutrient Distribution Ranges (AMDR) for adults:

Carbs: 45–65% of your daily calories

Protein: 10–35% of your daily calories

Fat: 20–35% of your daily calories

The guidelines also recommend that adults get at least 130 grams of carbs per day. This is the Recommended Dietary Allowance (RDA) and considered the amount necessary to provide your brain with enough glucose.

If there isn't enough glucose available — which can happen if you're following a strict keto diet or have issues regulating your insulin levels due to conditions like diabetes — your body is able to get energy by breaking down fat and protein.

When it comes to protein, the RDA for adults is at least 0.36 grams per pound (0.8 grams per kg) of body weight.

Keep in mind, though, that the appropriate amount of macronutrients for each person varies based on their age, activity levels, sex, and other circumstances.

For example, children and adolescents may need more calories from fat than adults do for proper brain development.

Older adults, on the other hand, need more protein to preserve muscle mass. Many experts recommend a protein intake of at least 0.45–0.54 grams per pound (1.0–1.2 grams per kg) for adults over the age of 65.

Athletes and highly active people often need more carbs and protein than those who are less active. They should aim for the higher end of the recommended ranges. Extra protein supports muscle building after exercise, while carbs provide calories to replenish energy stores.

If you're trying to lose weight, you might benefit from eating slightly below the recommended range of calories from carbs and above the range recommended for protein. Extra protein can help you feel full, while fewer carbs can promote a calorie deficit.

2

THE BENEFITS OF A HIGH PROTEIN DIET

Increasing your protein intake may help promote weight loss in many different ways.

Appetite and fullness

Protein increases the production of hormones like PYY and GLP-1, both of which help you feel full and satisfied. A 2020 review   also found that protein reduces levels of ghrelin, known as the "hunger hormone."

These effects of a high protein intake could lead to a natural reduction in food intake.

Metabolic rate

A 2018 review found that higher protein intake may boost your basal (BMR) and resting (RMM) metabolic rates. This can help you burn more calories for several hours after eating, as well as during your sleep.

Protein may also increase how much energy your body uses to absorb, metabolize, and store food. This is called the thermic effect of food (TEF). The TEF for protein is 20–30%, meaning that 20–30% of the calories found in protein are used simply to digest it. Meanwhile, the TEF for carbs and fat is 5–10% and 0–3%, respectively.

Body composition

Protein's ability to suppress appetite, promote fullness, and increase your metabolism can help you lose weight.

A 2020 review found that increasing protein intake promotes weight and fat loss while retaining muscle mass. The authors also note that high protein intake has long-term weight loss benefits and could help prevent weight regain.

Typically, when you reduce your calorie intake, your metabolism slows down. This is partly due to muscle loss. However, a higher protein intake can help protect against muscle loss and keep your metabolic rate up.

Boosts calorie burn

You burn more calories by eating protein because your body has to work harder to chew and digest the food. This is known as the thermic effect of food.

You may be more inclined to choose nutrient-dense foods

When you plan a meal around a lean source of protein, you have less space on your plate for less nutritious foods. Learning to eat different types of protein may also improve your diet. If you eat tuna, for example, you benefit from the fish's protein and healthy fats.

You'll build and maintain more muscle mass

A strong body performs better throughout daily activities, and muscles also burn more calories than fat, even at rest.

Different sources of high-quality protein and their nutritional profiles

Well-rounded high-protein diets often emphasize lean protein, nutrient-packed vegetables and berries, and whole grains. It's important to consider a wide range of protein sources. This may include animal and plant-based foods, including:

- Lean cuts of red meat (sirloin tip, top round, filet mignon)
- 75–80% lean ground beef
- Chicken breasts and thighs
- Seafood filets (salmon, cod, halibut)
- Beans (black, pinto, kidney)

- Vegetables (dark leafy greens, peppers, mushrooms, broccoli, cauliflower)
- Soy milk
- Low-fat milk, cheeses, and yogurt
- Eggs
- Nuts and seeds (almonds, walnuts, chia seeds, hemp seeds)
- Berries (blueberries, strawberries, and raspberries)
- Whole grains (quinoa, amaranth, barley)

Prioritizing foods like:

Poultry (chicken and turkey breast, egg whites) seafood (shrimp, tuna, and halibut) is essential as they are much higher in protein content.

Practical tips for incorporating more protein into meals and snacks

Any nutritious diet for weight loss or wellness should include a balance of the three macronutrients (or macros): fat, carbohydrates, and protein. A high-protein diet contains at least 20% of calories from protein. The amount of protein you should eat depends on a few factors, including age, gender, body size, and activity level.

General guidelines advise getting 10% to 35% of your total calories from protein. Active adults may require 1.2 to 1.7 grams (g) per kilogram (kg) of body weight per day. This equates to 82 to 116 grams for a person weighing 150 pounds. The official recommended daily allowance (RDA) for healthy adults is a minimum of 0.8 g/kg/day, which equates to 54 grams of protein for a person who weighs 150 pounds.

Use a food diary app or website to help you establish, track, and maintain your protein values and goals

A typical starting ratio for a high-protein diet is 30% of calories from protein, 30% from fat, and 40% from carbohydrates. But a starting ratio is just that—a starting point. Many proponents of high-protein diets find they do better with a little more or a little less of a macronutrient, which means you can adjust your macros as needed while maintaining a high-protein approach.

Following a high-protein diet typically requires:

Including protein at every meal

Planning meals around a protein, such as lean beef, chicken, or pork, and filling the rest of the plate with vegetables.

Skipping processed carbs

Instead of eating refined grains, like white rice, pasta, and bread, include small portions of whole grains that are high in protein, like amaranth or quinoa; or replace pasta with spiraled zucchini or carrots and substitute riced cauliflower for white rice.

Snacking on protein

Keeping high-protein snacks like almonds, Greek yogurt, hummus, ricotta cheese, and string cheese on hand for when between-meal hunger strikes.

Starting your day with protein

Focusing on high-protein breakfast foods like eggs and smoothies made with protein powder, such as whey, pea protein, or collagen.

Sample meal plans and recipes featuring high-protein foods

Each meal on a high-protein diet features a serving of protein accompanied by vegetables and smaller servings of certain fruits and whole grains. You can also snack on protein in between meals to curb hunger. Nuts or low-fat string cheese are great options.

Here's a sample menu that provides about 100 g of protein per day. You can choose to accompany these meals with water or a glass of wine at dinner. Keep in mind that if you decide to follow this diet, other meals may be more appropriate to suit your tastes and preferences.

Monday

Breakfast: 3 eggs, 1 slice whole grain toast with 1 tablespoon almond butter, and 1 pear.

Lunch: Fresh avocado and cottage cheese salad and an orange.

Dinner: 6 ounces (oz) (170 g) steak, sweet potato and grilled zucchini.

Tuesday

Breakfast: Smoothie made with 1 scoop protein powder, 1 cup coconut milk, and strawberries.

Lunch: 4 oz (114 g) canned salmon, mixed greens, olive oil and vinegar, and an apple.

Dinner: 4 oz (114 g) grilled chicken with quinoa and Brussels sprouts.

Wednesday

Breakfast: Oatmeal and 1 cup plain Greek yogurt with 1/4 cup chopped pecans.

Lunch: 4 oz (114 g) chicken mixed with 1 avocado, red bell pepper, and peach.

Dinner: Turkey pumpkin chili and brown rice.

Thursday

Breakfast: Omelet made with 3 eggs, 1 oz cheese, chili peppers, black olives and salsa, and an orange.

Lunch: Leftover turkey pumpkin chili and brown rice.

Dinner: 4 oz (114 g) halibut, lentils, and broccoli.

Friday

Breakfast: 1 cup cottage cheese with 1/4 cup chopped walnuts, diced apples, and cinnamon.

Lunch: 4 oz (114 g) canned salmon mixed with healthy mayo on sprouted grain bread, and carrot sticks.

Dinner: Chicken meatballs with marinara sauce, spaghetti squash, and raspberries.

Saturday

Breakfast: Frittata made with 3 eggs, 1 oz cheese, and 1/2 cup diced potatoes.

Lunch: Leftover chicken meatballs with marinara sauce and spaghetti squash with an apple.

Dinner: Fajitas with 3 oz (85 g) shrimp, grilled onions, bell peppers, guacamole, and 1/2 cup black beans on a corn tortilla.

Sunday

Breakfast: Protein pumpkin pancakes topped with 1/4 cup chopped pecans.

Lunch: 1 cup plain Greek yogurt mixed with 1/4 cup chopped mixed nuts and pineapple.

Dinner: 6 oz (170 g) grilled salmon, with potatoes and sautéed spinach.

Some high protein snacks can also help you boost your protein intake and promote weight loss

3

HARNESSING THE POWER OF FIBER FOR WEIGHT LOSS

Dietary fiber, or just fiber, describes the type of carbohydrates in food that our bodies can't digest. We can find fiber in a wide variety of different fruits, vegetables, grains, and seeds, and there are two main types — soluble fiber and insoluble fiber.

Eating fiber is one of the many ways that we nourish our gut, but research has shown that there are even more benefits to eating a high fiber diet. Below, we'll explore some of those benefits, and share how you can get more high fiber foods onto your plate and into your gut.

The health benefits of dietary fiber

Here are 10 of fiber's health benefits to encourage you to get your fill:

1. Healthy Weight Loss

It is well-known increasing your dietary fiber intake may help in your weight loss journey. In a 2019 randomized controlled trial published in The Journal of Nutrition, participants were assigned to one of four different calorie-restricted groups. They were also instructed to increase their dietary fiber intake at various intervals and to include 90 minutes of physical activity each week. Results showed that regardless of diet type, participants lost about the same amount of weight. Study authors felt this was due to the fiber intake and not calorie consumption, which affirms what previous studies had shown—that increasing your fiber intake can help you lose weight.

Fiber-rich foods fill you up faster and keep you satisfied longer.

2. Weight Control

While more research needs to be performed, there is some evidence that suggests that those who eat more fiber tend to be leaner, according to a 2023 study in Frontiers in Nutrition. Researchers found that people who ate the most fiber after losing weight weighed less than those who ate less dietary fiber.

3. Lower Type 2 Diabetes Risk

A 2020 study published in the Journal of Diabetes Investigation found that a higher overall intake of dietary fiber was associated with a lower risk of type 2 diabetes. And while some previous studies showed that insoluble fiber was best type of fiber for lowering type 2 diabetes risk, this study suggests that the combination of soluble and insoluble fiber predicted greater prevention of type 2 diabetes. While it's not totally clear why fiber cuts type 2 diabetes risk, the researchers believe that it could be a combination of fiber's favorable effect on blood glucose levels, creating a healthier gut microbiome and lowering inflammation in the body that may help stave off the development of diabetes.

4. Lower Odds of Heart Disease

According to a 2022 BMC Public Health study, a higher fiber intake was associated with a reduced risk for cardiovascular disease (CVD) in a large group of Americans. Researchers don't completely understand how fiber works, but they think that soluble fiber plays a role in decreasing lipid uptake from the intestinal tract, resulting in lower blood levels of cholesterol according to a 2023 Advances in Nutrition review. In addition, experts say that dietary fiber reduces inflammation which can result in CVD in a 2022 JAMA Network Open article.

5. Increased Beneficial Gut Bacteria

The good bacteria that make up your gut's microbiome feed off fiber which helps them flourish. According to a 2022 review article in Animal Nutrition, as your gut bacteria gobble up fiber that has fermented in your GI tract, they produce short-chain fatty acids that have a host of benefits—including lowering systemic inflammation, which has been linked to many chronic health problems.

When you increase your fiber intake, it doesn't take long to see the results. You can start to see the changes in gut bacteria within just a few days. The catch: You've got to consistently get enough grams of fiber over time to keep getting the benefits. Skimping on fiber shifts bacteria populations that may have negative consequences and result in increased inflammation in the body.

6. Reduced Risk of Certain Cancers

While studies are mixed, most seem to point to higher fiber consumption lowering the risk of cancer, especially colorectal and breast cancers. For example, in a 2020 review in The American Journal of Clinical Nutrition, researchers found that higher fiber intake, in particular, the fiber found in whole grains, was correlated with a reduced risk of colorectal cancer. And another 2020 review published in Cancer found that soluble fiber and fruit fiber had the strongest associations with reduced risk of breast cancer. This falls in line with the American Cancer Society's recommendations to eat foods rich in total fiber, which include fruits, vegetables and whole grains.

7. Longer Life

A 2022 review in the Journal of Translational Medicine found that people who ate enough total fiber—which includes soluble and insoluble fibers—had a lower chance of dying early from anything, including cardiovascular disease and cancer. This means that even if you were to get heart disease, cancer or another condition, consuming enough fiber may protect you from dying from it.

8. More Regular Bowel Movements

If you find yourself constipated, fiber might help. Fiber makes your poop softer and bulkier—both of which speed its passage from your body. But different types of fiber may provide varying levels of success in your quest for more regular bowel movements. A 2020 review in the Journal of the American Association of Nurse Practitioners suggests that psyllium fiber beats out other types of fiber for those with chronic idiopathic constipation, which is characterized by difficult, infrequent or incomplete bowel movements. Other studies, like the 2021 review in Clinical and Experimental Gastroenterology note that including plenty of water with your high-fiber diet also helps move things along in your gut better than fiber alone.

9. All-Natural Detox

Fiber naturally scrubs and promotes the elimination of toxins from your GI tract. Soluble fiber soaks up potentially harmful compounds, such as excess estrogen and unhealthy fats, before they can be absorbed by the body. And because insoluble fiber makes things move along more quickly, it limits the amount of time that chemicals like BPA, mercury and pesticides stay in your system. The faster they go through you, the less chance they have to cause harm.

10. Strong Bones

Some types of soluble fiber—known as prebiotics—have been shown to contribute to a greater bioavailability of minerals, like calcium, in your colon. The increase in bioavailability supports maintain bone density, according to a 2018 review in the journal Calcified Tissue International. Prebiotics provide food for your beneficial gut bacteria and can be found in certain fruits, vegetables, nuts and whole grains, such as asparagus, bananas, walnuts, onions, legumes, wheat and oats.

Types of dietary fiber

Fiber is commonly classified as soluble, which dissolves in water, or insoluble, which doesn't dissolve.

Soluble fiber: This type of fiber dissolves in water to form a gel-like material. It can help lower blood cholesterol and glucose levels. Soluble fiber is found in oats, peas, beans, apples, citrus fruits, carrots, barley and psyllium.

Insoluble fiber: This type of fiber promotes the movement of material through your digestive system and increases stool bulk, so it can be of benefit to those who struggle with constipation or irregular stools. Whole-wheat flour, wheat bran, nuts, beans and vegetables, such as cauliflower, green beans and potatoes, are good sources of insoluble fiber.

The amount of soluble and insoluble fiber varies in different plant foods. To receive the greatest health benefit, eat a wide variety of high-fiber foods.

There is also a lot of overlap between soluble and insoluble fibers. Some insoluble fibers can be digested by the good bacteria in the intestine, and most foods contain both soluble and insoluble fibers.

Health authorities recommend that men and women eat 38 and 25 grams of fiber per day, respectively.

Foods rich in fiber and how to incorporate them into a daily diet

What foods are most high in fiber?

You've probably already been eating foods that are high in fiber. But just in case — here are a few of our top picks for high fiber foods to add to your plate.

Lentils

20.5 grams of fiber per cup, uncooked

10.7 grams of fiber in every 100 grams

Lentils are a great source of nutrients and an even better source of dietary fiber. Just 1 cup of uncooked lentils nets over 20 grams of fiber, which makes them great for batch recipes like curries, stews, and soups.

Oats

16.5 grams of fiber per cup, uncooked

10.6 grams of fiber in every 100 grams

Oats are another quick, easy, and affordable source of dietary fiber, especially for breakfast. But even if you're not a fan of oats in the morning, you can still use them in other baking recipes, like breads, muffins, and more.

Black beans

15 grams of fiber per cup, cooked

8.7 grams of fiber in every 100 grams

Black beans are a staple in plant-based diets because they're not just high in fiber — they're also a great source of protein. One cup of cooked black beans has 15 grams of fiber, which is around half the recommended daily amount.

Kidney beans

13.1 grams of fiber per cup, cooked

7.4 grams of fiber in every 100 grams

Like black beans, kidney beans are also high in vitamins, minerals, protein, and fiber. Kidney beans are versatile and can be found in a variety of recipes, like vegetarian chili, red beans and rice, and even cold salads.

Chickpeas

12.5 grams of fiber per cup, cooked

7.6 grams of fiber in every 100 grams

Chickpeas are another great plant-based source of protein and dietary fiber. And you might be surprised by all the ways you can eat them — in soups, stews, salads, curries, and even roasted in the oven for a crunchy snack.

Avocado

10 grams of fiber per cup

6.7 grams of fiber in every 100 grams

Avocados are deliciously creamy and nutrient-dense — with plenty of fiber, too. Most people enjoy avocados on toast or in salads, but if you're looking for a little extra fiber in the morning, they also taste great in smoothies.

Chia seeds

9.75 grams of fiber per ounce, dried

34.4 grams of fiber in every 100 grams

Chia seeds are one of the best sources of soluble fiber, the type of fiber that helps slow down digestion and balance blood sugar. If you want to add chia seeds to your diet, your body will process them easier if you soak them first.

Raspberries

8 grams of fiber per cup

6.5 grams of fiber in every 100 grams

Raspberries may seem like a sweet treat, but did you know that they're also high in fiber? Adding 1 cup of these berries to your breakfast or a snack will net you 8 grams of fiber, getting you that much closer to your fiber goal.

Strategies for increasing fiber intake without feeling deprived

Below are tips for fitting in more fiber:

Jump-start your day

For breakfast choose a high-fiber breakfast cereal — 5 or more grams of fiber a serving. Opt for cereals with "whole grain," "bran" or "fiber" in the name. Or add a few tablespoons of unprocessed wheat bran to your favorite cereal.

Switch to whole grains

Consume at least half of all grains as whole grains. Look for breads that list whole wheat, whole-wheat flour or another whole grain as the first ingredient on the label and have at least 2 grams of dietary fiber a serving. Experiment with brown rice, wild rice, barley, whole-wheat pasta and bulgur wheat.

Bulk up baked goods

Substitute whole-grain flour for half or all of the white flour when baking. Try adding crushed bran cereal, unprocessed wheat bran or uncooked oatmeal to muffins, cakes and cookies.

Lean on legumes

Beans, peas and lentils are excellent sources of fiber. Add kidney beans to canned soup or a green salad. Or make nachos with refried black beans, lots of fresh veggies, whole-wheat tortilla chips and salsa.

Eat more fruit and vegetables

Fruits and vegetables are rich in fiber, as well as vitamins and minerals. Try to eat five or more servings daily.

Make snacks count

Fresh fruits, raw vegetables, low-fat popcorn and whole-grain crackers are all good choices. A handful of nuts or dried fruits also is a healthy, high-fiber snack — although be aware that nuts and dried fruits are high in calories.

High-fiber foods are good for your health. But adding too much fiber too quickly can promote intestinal gas, abdominal bloating and cramping. Increase fiber in your diet gradually over a few weeks. This allows the natural bacteria in your digestive system to adjust to the change.

Also, drink plenty of water. Fiber works best when it absorbs water, making your stool soft and bulky.

4

CRAFTING LOW-CALORIE MEALS WITHOUT SACRIFICING FLAVOR

Put simply, calorie density is the number of calories within a particular food in relation to its weight or volume. You'll likely see a food's calorie density measured as calories per 100g (or 3.5 oz if you're looking at an imperial measurement). You might also see it referred to as energy density.

Different foods have different calorie densities. For example, tomatoes have about 18 calories per 100g, wholemeal pasta has 149 calories per 100g, and olive oil has around 884 calories per 100g. This makes tomatoes the least calorie-dense food out of the 3 and olive oil the most calorie dense.

The reason is that foods with high water content (such as tomatoes) typically have a lower calorie density, while fat (which olive oil contains a lot of) is the most calorie-dense macronutrient. It has about 9 calories per gram (900 calories per 100g) whereas carbs and protein both contain 4 calories per gram (400 calories per 100g)

Choosing foods with a low-calorie density can help with weight loss. It makes you automatically eat fewer calories while still eating large and filling portions.

An easier way to make sense of this is to imagine a full plate of food. The fewer calories the plate contains, the lower the calorie density of the meal.

A vegetable with 30 calories per 100 grams has a low-calorie density, while chocolate with 550 calories per 100 grams has a very high-calorie density.

Although calorie density may be less known than other weight management concepts like calorie counting, choosing foods based on this measure may be more straightforward and effective.

For example, basing your diet on low-calorie-density foods limits you to predominantly healthy and nutrient-rich whole foods.

It can quickly clean up your diet, eliminating most calorie-dense, processed foods that are generally unhealthy and easy to overeat.

How do you calculate calorie density?

If you're buying a bag of rice or a carton of milk, it's easy to work out its calorie density. You'll see it in the nutrition panel, usually given per serve and per 100g.

But if you're eating something that doesn't come out of a packet, like fresh fruit and veg, you might have a little more trouble uncovering its nutritional information. Instead, you can calculate its calorie density by dividing the number of calories per serving by the serving size.

Let's use grapes as an example. One cup of grapes is generally considered one serving. In grams, that's about 150g. A single serving of grapes has about 104 calories. If we divide 104 by 150, we can work out that the energy density per gram is 0.69 calories and the energy density per 100g is 69 calories (0.69 x 100).

Compare this to tomatoes, which contain 18 calories per 100g and whole-meal pasta, which has about 149 calories per 100g, and we can see that grapes sit somewhere in between.

Calorie density measures the calorie content of food relative to its weight or volume.

It is also called energy density and is usually measured as calories per 3.5 ounces (100 grams) of food.

What role does calorie density play in weight loss?

So, what's the advantage of understanding calorie density? Well, if you know the difference between the energy density of different foods, you can opt for things that are high in nutrition but lower in calories — potentially helping you to lose weight.

We know that eating too many high-calorie, low-nutrition foods can lead to weight gain. That's simply because they give your body a lot of energy in small portion sizes, meaning they don't really fill you up. Plus, research shows they're quite easy to overeat.

On the other hand, low calorie density foods can make you feel fuller because you're able to eat bigger portions without consuming as many calories.

This is why calorie density is preferable to simply calorie counting. If you're counting calories, you might hit your daily calorie limit by only eating a few pizza slices and a block of chocolate — and still end up hungry. But if you eat a bowl of porridge, a salad sandwich on whole-meal bread, and a plate of roast chicken with veggies, you might very well consume a similar number of calories but feel much more satisfied.

The other advantage is that many low calorie density foods tend to be more nutritious. Healthier foods like vegetables, fruits, whole grains, and legumes are on the lower end when it comes to calorie density, while oils, meats, cheese, sweets, and processed foods are on the higher end.

Lower calorie-density foods are also higher in fibre, which takes longer to digest and keeps you fuller for longer — meaning you're more inclined to eat less.

There have been several studies done on the relationship between calorie density and weight, too. Research shows that eating a high-energy-density diet is closely linked to obesity and a higher waist circumference, as well as related conditions like insulin resistance and metabolic disorders. By contrast, lower energy density diets are connected to lower amounts of abdominal fat

The difference between calorie density and nutrient density

You may also have heard of a concept known as 'nutrient density' in relation to food.

Rather than being a measure of how many calories are in a specific weight of food, nutrient density refers to the amount of nutrients a food provides relative to its calorie content. Foods with a high nutrient density are usually referred to as being nutrient-dense. This means they pack a real nutritional punch for the number of calories they contain.

Many low calorie density foods — such as vegetables, fruit, and whole grains — also happen to be nutrient-dense foods because they offer vitamins, minerals, complex carbs, and other things that are good for your body.

Foods that have a low-calorie density

Most natural foods have a very low-calorie density. These include:

Vegetables: Most green vegetables have the lowest calorie density of all foods because they're primarily made up of water, fiber, and a very small number of carbs.

Meat and fish: Lean proteins like chicken, white fish, and turkey have a low-calorie density, yet fattier meats and fish have a moderate to high density.

Fruits: These have a low-calorie density because of their high fiber and water content. Berries and other watery fruits tend to have the lowest density.

Milk and yogurt: Reduced-fat milk and yogurts with no added sugar also have a low-calorie density and provide a good source of protein.

Eggs: Whole eggs are a protein-packed superfood with a moderate calorie density, especially when combined with vegetables.

Starchy carbs: Some natural starchy carbs like potatoes, legumes, and other root vegetables have low-calorie density. This is especially true once cooked, as they fill with water.

Sugar-free drinks: These beverages, such as water, coffee, and tea, have a low-calorie density and can help keep you full.

There is no reason to eliminate high-fat foods completely. Just keep your intake moderate. Many healthy high-fat foods, such as nuts, avocados, and olive oil, may contribute to weight gain if you eat too many.

High-calorie-density foods to limit

If you want to try this approach and base your food selection on calorie density, you will need to limit your intake of foods with high-calorie density, including:

Candy and chips: Candy and chips are high in sugar and fat, making them very calorie-dense and easy to overeat.

Pastries and cakes: Like candy, pastries and cakes are very calorie-dense and easy to overeat.

Fast foods: These are some of the most calorie-dense foods available. Studies show that a fast food meal packs around twice the calories of a regular, healthy meal.

Oils: While certain oils, such as coconut and olive oil, are healthy, they still have a very high-calorie density. Consume healthy oils in moderation.

High-fat dairy: Foods like butter, cream, and cheese have very high-calorie densities. Consume them in moderation.

Fatty meats: Some fatty meats have a very high-calorie density. These include bacon, sausages, lamb, and fatty beef cuts.

Nuts: Like other healthy fat sources, nuts are very calorie-dense. While they do have many health benefits, they're easy to overeat. Try measuring out your portions before you eat them.

High-fat condiments: Some sauces and condiments, such as mayonnaise, pesto, and ranch dressing, are very high in calories and should mostly be avoided.

Sugary drinks: Some smoothies and full-fat milkshakes are high in calories and should be avoided as much as possible.

Techniques for reducing calories while still enjoying satisfying meals

Let's explore subtle adjustments that can yield significant benefits for both your health and your taste buds:

Opt for Greek Yogurt over Sour Cream

While sour cream adds richness to savory dishes, it also packs a caloric punch. Switching to lower-fat Greek yogurt can halve the calories while adding a protein boost to keep you satisfied longer. Greek yogurt offers over one hundred times more protein per gram than sour cream, making it a superior choice for dips, dressings, baked potato toppings, and more.

Sauté with Broth Instead of Oil

When sautéing vegetables or cooking grains like rice or quinoa, swap out oil for low-sodium vegetable or chicken broth. This simple switch dramatically reduces calories, as one tablespoon of oil contains 120 calories compared to less than 10 calories in one cup of broth. You'll still achieve that delightful sautéed flavor, and for added richness, finish with a touch of butter or opt for a healthy oil like olive oil.

Bulk Up Casseroles with Vegetables

To boost nutrition and cut calories in creamy casseroles, increase the vegetable content. Chopped spinach, kale, broccoli, carrots, mushrooms, and other veggies not only add fiber and nutrients but also displace heavier ingredients. By finely chopping or pureeing the vegetables, you seamlessly incorporate them into the dish, elevating its health profile without sacrificing taste.

Use Cauliflower Rice Instead of Grains

Replace rice and other grains with cauliflower rice for a lower-calorie, lower-carb alternative. With only twenty-seven calories per cup compared to 216 calories in white rice, cauliflower rice allows you to enjoy hearty meals with significantly fewer calories. Its versatility shines in stir-fries, fajitas, under saucy dishes, and more, absorbing flavors splendidly while keeping your meals light.

Swap Greek Yogurt for Mayo

Substitute full-fat mayonnaise with creamy Greek yogurt for a healthier option in recipes like chicken or tuna salad, dressings, sandwich spreads, and dips. Greek yogurt provides a rich texture with substantially fewer calories and less fat per tablespoon compared to mayo, making it a guilt-free choice for indulgent dishes.

Opt for Zoodles Instead of Pasta

For a low-carb, low-calorie alternative to pasta, try spiralized zucchini noodles or "zoodles" in your favorite pasta dishes. With approximately 20 calories per cup, zoodles significantly reduce calorie intake compared to traditional pasta while seamlessly integrating into various recipes, from pasta bakes to casseroles.

Puree Canned Beans for Dips and Spreads

Harness the protein and fiber of canned beans by transforming them into dips, spreads, and more. White beans, chickpeas, black beans, or any variety can be pureed into creamy textures that substitute for high-calorie ingredients like sour cream, mayo, or cream cheese. Experiment with spices and herbs to create versatile dips, spreads, and sauces that enhance both flavor and nutrition.

Make Smart Ingredient Substitutions

You don't have to give up your favorite comfort foods to eat healthier. With simple swaps and adjustments, you can give indulgent dishes a healthy makeover without sacrificing flavor. Enjoy familiar textures and tastes while reducing calories and increasing nutritional value. Small changes can yield significant results, allowing you to savor beloved classics guilt-free.

In essence, healthy eating doesn't mean deprivation; it's about creativity and flexibility with ingredients. Expand your culinary repertoire with healthier versions of your favorite dishes, allowing you to indulge in comfort food while nourishing your body and soul.

Creating balanced, nutrient-dense meals that support weight loss goals

Creating a calorie deficit in a nutrient-dense way

All weight loss plans have one thing in common — they get you to eat fewer calories than you burn

However, though a calorie deficit will help you lose weight regardless of how it's created, what you eat is just as important as how much you eat. That's because the food choices you make are instrumental in helping you meet your nutrient needs.

A good weight loss meal plan should follow some universal criteria:

Includes plenty of protein and fiber: Protein- and fiber-rich foods help keep you fuller for longer, reducing cravings and helping you feel satisfied with smaller portions.

Limits processed foods and added sugar: Rich in calories yet low in nutrients, these foods fail to stimulate fullness centers in your brain and make it difficult to lose weight or meet your nutrient needs (9, 10).

Includes a variety of fruits and vegetables: Both are rich in water and fiber, contributing to feelings of fullness. These nutrient-rich foods also make it easier to meet your daily nutrient requirements.

Building nutrient-dense meals

To incorporate these tips into your weight loss meal plan, start by filling one-third to one-half of your plate with non-starchy vegetables. These are low in calories and provide water, fiber, and many of the vitamins and minerals you need.

Then, fill one-quarter to one-third of your plate with protein-rich foods, such as meat, fish, tofu, seitan, or legumes, and the remainder with whole grains, fruit, or starchy vegetables. These add protein, vitamins, minerals, and more fiber.

You can boost the flavor of your meal with a dash of healthy fats from foods like avocados, olives, nuts, and seeds.

Some people may benefit from having a snack to tide their hunger over between meals. Protein- and fiber-rich snacks seem the most effective for weight loss.

Good examples include apple slices with peanut butter, vegetables and hummus, roasted chickpeas, or Greek yogurt with fruit and nuts.

5

HIGH PROTEIN RECIPES YOU MUST TRY!

DELIGHTFUL RECIPES FOR BREAKFAST

High protein breakfast

Ingredients

15ml olive oil

130g tomatoes, halved

4 rashers turkey bacon

180g sirloin steak, trimmed of visible fat

150g mushrooms, sliced

160g spinach

1 egg

Instructions

STEP 1

Heat grill to high. Drizzle a little of the oil on your tomatoes and season well. Lay the tomatoes on a baking tray lined with foil and place under the grill. Cook for 4-5 mins, then add the bacon to the tray. Turn the bacon as necessary until it is cooked through. Turn off the grill and shut the door to keep everything warm.

STEP 2

Meanwhile, heat the remaining oil in a large, non-stick frying pan over a high heat. Season your steak well and, when the pan is very hot, fry for 3-4 mins each side for medium-rare, then leave it to rest until you are ready to eat.

STEP 3

While the steak is resting, throw the mushrooms into the still-hot pan, fry for 2-3 mins until browned, then move to one side of the pan. Add the spinach to the other side of the pan and cook until wilted. Put a saucepan of water on to boil.

STEP 4

Crack the egg into the boiling water, then reduce the heat until the water is gently simmering. Poach the egg for 3-4 mins or until the white has set but the yolk is still runny. Carefully lift it out with a slotted spoon and drain on kitchen paper. Serve everything together and top with the poached egg.

Easy protein pancakes

Ingredients

1 banana

75g oats

3 large eggs

2 tbsp milk (dairy, soya, oat or nut milks all work)

1 tbsp baking powder

pinch of cinnamon

2 tbsp protein powder (whey, pea or whatever your preference)

coconut oil, or a flavourless oil, for frying

nut butter, maple syrup and berries or sliced banana to serve

Instructions

STEP 1

Whizz the banana, oats, eggs, milk, baking powder, cinnamon and protein powder in a blender for 1-2 mins until smooth. Check the oats have broken down, if not, blend for another minute.

STEP 2

Heat a drizzle of oil in a pan. Pour or ladle in 2-3 rounds of batter, leaving a little space between each to spread. Cook for 1-2 minutes, until bubbles start to appear on the surface and the underside is golden. Flip over and cook for another minute until cooked through. Transfer to a warmed oven and repeat with the remaining batter. Serve in stacks with nut butter, maple syrup and fruit.

Healthy pepper, tomato & ham omelette

Ingredients

2 whole eggs and 3 egg whites

1 tsp olive oil

1 red pepper, deseeded and finely chopped

2 spring onions, white and green parts kept separate, and finely chopped

few slices wafer-thin extra-lean ham, shredded

25g reduced-fat mature cheddar

wholemeal toast, to serve (optional)

1-2 chopped fresh tomatoes, to serve (optional)

Instructions

STEP 1

Mix the eggs and egg whites with some seasoning and set aside. Heat the oil in a medium non-stick frying pan and cook the pepper for 3-4 mins. Throw in the white parts of the spring onions and cook for 1 min more. Pour in the eggs and cook over a medium heat until almost completely set.

STEP 2

Sprinkle on the ham and cheese, and continue cooking until just set in the centre, or flash it under a hot grill if you like it more well done. Serve straight from the pan with the green part of the spring onions sprinkled on top, the chopped tomato and some wholemeal toast, if you like.

Protein pancakes with banana

Ingredients

3 eggs

75g porridge oats

1 large, ripe banana

2 tbsp protein powder, any kind

2 tbsp milk, any kind

1 tbsp baking powder

¼ tsp ground cinnamon

neutral oil, for the pan

To serve

Greek yogurt, sliced bananas and maple syrup

Instructions

STEP 1

Tip the eggs, oats, banana protein powder, milk, baking powder and cinnamon into a blender and blitz for 1-2 mins until smooth. Check the oats have broken down, if not, blitz for another minute.

STEP 2

Heat a drizzle of oil in a pan. Pour or ladle in 2-3 rounds of batter, leaving a little space between each to spread. Cook for 1-2 mins until bubbles start to appear on the surface and the underside is golden. Flip over and cook for another minute until cooked through. Transfer to a warmed oven and repeat with the remaining batter.

STEP 3

Serve topped with a dollop of Greek yogurt, sliced bananas and maple syrup.

Avocado & black bean eggs

Ingredients

2 tsp rapeseed oil

1 red chilli, deseeded and thinly sliced

1 large garlic clove, sliced

2 large eggs

400g can black beans

½ x 400g can cherry tomatoes

¼ tsp cumin seeds

1 small avocado, halved and sliced

handful fresh, chopped coriander

1 lime, cut into wedges

Instructions

STEP 1

Heat the oil in a large non-stick frying pan. Add the chilli and garlic and cook until softened and starting to colour. Break in the eggs on either side of the pan. Once they start to set, spoon the beans (with their juice) and the tomatoes around the pan and sprinkle over the cumin seeds. You're aiming to warm the beans and tomatoes rather than cook them.

STEP 2

Remove the pan from the heat and scatter over the avocado and coriander. Squeeze over half of the lime wedges. Serve with the remaining wedges on the side for squeezing over.

Vegan protein pancakes

Ingredients

For the batter

2 tbsp ground flaxseeds

20g ground almonds

300ml soya milk

200g quinoa flour

1 medium banana, mashed

2 tbsp maple syrup

coconut oil, for frying

For the blueberry chia jam (makes 200ml)

200g blueberries, mashed

2 tbsp chia seeds

1-2 tbsp maple syrup, to taste

2 tsp lemon juice

For the stack

100g coconut yogurt or Greek yogurt

1 tbsp pistachio nuts or pumpkin seeds, chopped, toasted if you like

2 tsp hulled hemp seeds

mixed berries

Instructions

STEP 1

In a small bowl stir the flaxseeds with 6 tbsp water and set aside to soak while you make the jam.

STEP 2

Mash the blueberries with a fork in a pan then set over a low-medium heat until syrupy and bubbling. Remove from the heat and stir in the chia seeds, maple syrup and lemon juice. Leave to cool slightly then transfer to a small serving jar.

STEP 3

Put the ground almonds, milk, flour, banana, maple syrup and a pinch of salt in a blender. Stir the flax to make sure it has become thick and gloopy, like an egg, then tip into the mix and blitz until smooth and thick.

STEP 4

Heat 1 tsp of coconut oil in a large frying pan over a medium heat and add tablespoon dollops of batter into the pan. Cook for a couple of mins on one side until the edges are browning, and bubbles have formed on top. Once the pale, white batter has turned a sandy colour, flip over with a spatula and cook for another few mins till dark golden brown. Set aside and keep warm while you repeat the process with the remaining batter, adding another tsp of coconut oil with each batch. You should make about 16 pancakes.

STEP 5

Pile the pancakes high between two plates, alternating the layers with spoonfuls of jam and yogurt. Dollop any remaining yogurt and another spoonful of jam on top then scatter over the nuts, seeds and berries to serve. Leftover jam will keep in the fridge for up to 1 week.

Egg foo yung

Ingredients

2 tbsp groundnut oil

150g protein of choice, such as raw king prawns (de-shelled and de-veined) or cooked chicken, cooked char siu pork or pre-fried tofu, cut into bite-sized pieces

1 small white onion, cut into strips

40g sliced mushrooms

40g peas

¼ tsp white pepper

4 eggs, whisked

Instructions

STEP 1

Heat a wok over a medium-high heat. Once hot, pour in the oil, then add your protein of choice and spread it out across the bottom of the wok. When it begins to brown, add the sliced onion and continue to cook for 1-2 mins, stirring regularly, to soften slightly. Tip in the mushrooms and stir.

STEP 2

When the mushrooms have started to soften, add the peas along with the white pepper and ½ tsp salt. Stir-fry for 1 min, then add the whisked eggs. Try not to stir the eggs – instead, pick up the wok and swirl the eggs around the rest of the Ingredients. Once they begin to set, slowly fold into the rest of the dish. Remove from the heat as soon as the eggs have nearly cooked all the way through.

DELIGHTFUL RECIPES FOR LUNCH

Bacon & mushroom pasta

Ingredients

400g penne (or other tube shape) pasta

250g pack chestnut or button mushrooms, wiped clean

8 rashers streaky bacon

4 tbsp pesto (fresh from the chiller cabinet if possible)

200ml carton 50% fat crème fraîche

handful basil leaves

Directions

STEP 1

Cook the pasta in boiling water in a large non-stick saucepan according to pack instructions. Meanwhile, slice the mushrooms and snip the bacon into bite-size pieces with scissors or a sharp knife.

STEP 2

Reserve a few drops of the cooking water in a cup or bowl, then drain the pasta and set aside. Fry the bacon and mushrooms in the same pan until golden, about 5 mins. Keep the heat high so the mushrooms fry in the bacon fat, rather than sweat.

STEP 3

Tip the pasta and reserved water back into the pan and stir over the heat for 1 min. Take the pan off the heat, spoon in the pesto and crème fraîche and most of the basil and stir to combine. Sprinkle with the remaining basil to serve.

Indian chickpeas with poached eggs

Ingredients

1 tbsp rapeseed oil

2 garlic cloves, chopped

1 yellow pepper, deseeded and diced

½ - 1 red chilli, deseeded and chopped

½ bunch spring onions (about 5), tops and whites sliced but kept separate

1 tsp cumin, plus a little extra to serve (optional)

1 tsp coriander

½ tsp turmeric

3 tomatoes, cut into wedges

⅓ pack coriander, chopped

400g can chickpeas in water, drained but liquid reserved

½ tsp reduced-salt bouillon powder (we used Marigold)

4 large eggs

Directions

STEP 1

Heat the oil in a non-stick sauté pan, add the garlic, pepper, chilli and the whites from the spring onions, and fry for 5 mins over a medium-high heat. Meanwhile, put a large pan of water on to boil.

STEP 2

Add the spices, tomatoes, most of the coriander and the chickpeas to the sauté pan and cook for 1-2 mins more. Stir in the bouillon powder and enough liquid from the chickpeas to moisten everything, and leave to simmer gently.

STEP 3

Once the water is at a rolling boil, crack in your eggs and poach for 2 mins, then remove with a slotted spoon. Stir the spring onion tops into the chickpeas, then very lightly crush a few of the chickpeas with a fork or potato masher. Spoon the chickpea mixture onto plates, scatter with the reserved coriander and top with the eggs. Serve with an extra sprinkle of cumin, if you like.

Air-fryer boiled eggs

Ingredients

6 eggs

toast, to serve (optional)

Directions

STEP 1

Heat the air-fryer to 180C. Put the eggs in the air-fryer basket and cook, in one layer, for 8-14 mins – nearer to 8 mins will be soft-boiled, while 14 mins will be hard-boiled.

STEP 2

Put the eggs in a bowl of ice cold water briefly to stop them from cooking. Peel or serve in egg cups with toast on the side, if you like.

Sausage pasta

Ingredients

1 tbsp olive oil

packet of 8 pork sausages (the best your budget will allow), cut into chunky pieces

1 large onion, chopped

2 garlic cloves, crushed

1 tsp chilli powder

400g can chopped tomatoes

300g short pasta such as fusilli or farfalle (just over half a 500g bag)

Directions

STEP 1

Put a large pan of water on to boil.

STEP 2

Heat 1 tbsp olive oil in a large frying pan and fry
chunky pieces of 8 pork sausages on a fairly high
heat until they are golden brown all over.

STEP 3

Now turn the heat down and add 1 large chopped
onion and 2 crushed garlic cloves, cooking them
until they have softened.

STEP 4

Stir in 1 tsp chilli powder and 400g chopped
tomatoes with the sausages, bring the sauce to the

boil then turn the heat down and let it bubble for about 10 minutes while you cook the pasta.

STEP 5

Drop 300g pasta into the pan of boiling water and cook according to the pack instructions.

STEP 6

Drain the pasta, then tip it into the frying pan with the sausage sauce, mixing well to coat. Dish up immediately with crusty bread.

Whole roasted salmon

Ingredients

1 x 2kg/4lb 8oz salmon, filleted to give two sides, skin on

1 lemon, sliced

good handful mixed herbs such as parsley, dill, chervil or tarragon

2 bay leaves

1-2 shallots, thinly sliced

splash white wine

Directions

STEP 1

Heat oven to 200C/180C fan/gas 6. Sit one of the salmon fillets, skin-side down, on a large sheet of foil or baking parchment. Scatter with the lemon slices, herbs, shallots and seasoning, then sit the second fillet on top – skin-side up. Tie in 2-3 places with string to secure, splash with wine and fold up the foil or paper to seal. Can be chilled for up to 3 hrs.

STEP 2

Place on a baking sheet and bake for 50 mins-1 hr until the salmon is cooked through – check by poking a knife into the fillets and making sure the flesh flakes easily. Serve in foil or paper on a serving plate, or carefully lift out using a couple of fish slices. Slice into portions and serve with the Lemon & chive mayonnaise and half-steamed broccoli.

Spanish rice & prawn one-pot

Ingredients

1 onion, sliced

1 red and 1 green pepper, deseeded and sliced

50g chorizo, sliced

2 garlic cloves, crushed

1 tbsp olive oil

250g easy cook basmati rice (we used Tilda)

400g can chopped tomato

200g raw, peeled prawns, defrosted if frozen

Directions

STEP 1

Boil the kettle. In a non-stick frying or shallow pan with a lid, fry the onion, peppers, chorizo and garlic in the oil over a high heat for 3 mins. Stir in the rice and chopped tomatoes with 500ml boiling water, cover, then cook over a high heat for 12 mins.

STEP 2

Uncover, then stir – the rice should be almost tender. Stir in the prawns, with a splash more water if the rice is looking dry, then cook for another min until the prawns are just pink and rice tender.

Greek lamb with smoked aubergine & minty broad beans

Ingredients

1 aubergine

zest and juice 0.5 lemon, plus wedges to serve

2 large garlic cloves, finely grated

1 tsp fresh oregano or 0.5 tsp dried

2 tsp extra virgin olive oil, plus 0.5 tsp

2 lean lamb leg steaks, about 100g/4oz each, all visible fat removed

100g (podded weight) baby broad beans, fresh or frozen

2 tbsp Greek bio yogurt

2 tsp tahini

12 mint leaves, roughly torn

Directions

STEP 1

Turn on your hob's largest gas flame and cook the aubergine directly over it for 7-8 mins, using tongs to turn it every 2 mins, until it is soft and the skin has charred. You can do this on the barbecue or under a hot grill if you don't have a gas hob. Allow to cool a little.

STEP 2

Mix the lemon zest, half the garlic, the oregano, some black pepper and 1/2 tsp oil, then use to coat the lamb steaks. Boil the broad beans for 4 mins.

STEP 3

Put the aubergine on a large plate and carefully remove and discard the skin. Use a knife and fork to finely chop the flesh, which should now be soft and pulpy. Tip into a bowl with the remaining garlic, the yogurt, tahini and some seasoning, and stir well.

STEP 4

Heat the griddle or barbecue and cook the lamb for 5 mins, turning once. Meanwhile, mix the beans with the lemon juice, remaining olive oil and the mint leaves. Spoon the aubergine purée onto plates and scatter round the minty beans. Top with the lamb and serve with lemon wedges.

DELIGHTFUL RECIPES FOR DINNER

Beef curry

Ingredients

2 tbsp oil

500g diced braising steak

1 tbsp butter

1 large onion, chopped

2 garlic cloves, crushed

1 thumb sized piece of ginger, finely grated

¼ tsp hot chilli powder

1 tsp turmeric

2 tsp ground coriander

3 cardamom pods, crushed

400g can chopped tomatoes

300ml beef stock

1 tsp sugar

2 tsp garam masala

2 tbsp double cream (optional)

½ small bunch coriander, roughly chopped

naan bread or rice, to serve

Directions

STEP 1

Heat one tbsp of the oil in a casserole pot over a medium-high heat. Season the beef and fry in the pot for 5-8 mins, turning with a pair of tongs half way until evenly browned. Set aside on a plate.

STEP 2

Heat the remaining oil and butter in the pan and add the onions. Fry gently for 15 mins or until golden brown and caramelised. Add the garlic, ginger, chilli, turmeric, ground coriander and cardamom and fry for two mins. Tip in the tomatoes, stock and sugar and bring to the simmer.

STEP 3

Add the beef, put a lid on top of the curry and cook over a low heat for 1 ½ – 2 hrs or until the meat is tender and falling apart. Remove the lid for the last 20 minutes of cooking.

STEP 4

Stir through the garam masala and cream (if using) and season to taste. Scatter over the coriander and serve with naan breads or rice.

Chicken tikka

Ingredients

3 large chicken breasts, cut into chunks

75g Greek yogurt

2 tbsp ginger and garlic paste

1 tbsp madras curry powder

1 tsp ground cumin

1 tsp ground coriander

1 tsp ground turmeric

1 tsp smoked paprika

2 tsp mild chilli powder

1 tbsp lemon juice

Directions

STEP 1

Tip all of the Ingredients into a large bowl with a big pinch of salt and pepper and mix well. Cover and chill for at least a few hours, but preferably overnight.

STEP 2

Heat the grill or a barbecue to high. Thread the chicken pieces onto four metal skewers, packing the pieces in so they're all touching. Put onto a baking tray under the grill, or onto the grills of the barbecue and cook for 4-5 mins, until charred, then flip and repeat.

Pulled chicken & black bean chilli

Ingredients

2 tbsp sunflower oil

2 onions, sliced

4 boneless, skinless chicken thighs

3 garlic cloves, finely chopped

1 tbsp oregano

1 tsp cumin seeds

3 tbsp chipotle in adobo or 1 tsp chipotle paste

350g passata

½ chicken stock shot or cube

400g can black beans, drained but not rinsed

½ lime, juiced

cooked rice or tortillas, coriander, feta, lime wedges and chopped red onion, to serve (optional)

Directions

STEP 1

Heat the oil in a shallow saucepan or casserole dish with a lid. Tip in the onions and cook over a medium-low heat for 5 mins until softened. Add the chicken and turn up the heat to medium. Stir in the garlic, a small pinch of sugar, the oregano, cumin seeds and some seasoning. Cook for a couple of minutes, then add the chipotle and cook for a few minutes more. Pour in the passata, 100ml water and add the stock. Season and bring to a simmer.

STEP 2

Cover with a lid and cook for 40-50 mins, stirring occasionally until the chicken is tender. Shred the chicken into the sauce using two forks, then stir through the beans. Simmer for 5 mins more, then turn off the heat. Squeeze in the lime juice. Can be kept chilled for three days and frozen for up to two months. Defrost thoroughly and reheat. Serve with rice or tortilla wraps, and some coriander, feta, lime wedges and red onion on the side, if you like.

Spicy cauliflower & halloumi rice

Ingredients

1 small head cauliflower (500g), broken into medium florets

150g baby spinach

1 tbsp rapeseed oil

1 red onion, sliced

120g halloumi, cut into cubes

1 garlic clove, crushed

1 thumb-sized piece ginger, finely grated

1 tsp ground turmeric

1 tbsp medium curry powder

2 x 250g pouches brown basmati rice

1 red chilli, finely sliced

Directions

STEP 1

Bring a large pan of salted water to the boil and
cook the cauliflower for 5 mins over a high heat,

adding the spinach for the final 2 mins. Drain and set aside.

STEP 2

Heat the oil in a large frying pan or shallow casserole dish and fry the onion over a medium heat for 5 mins. Turn up the heat, add the halloumi, cook for a further 5 mins, then add the garlic, ginger, turmeric and curry powder, and cook for 1 min more. Stir through the rice, cauliflower and spinach to warm everything through, adding 1 tbsp water if it looks a little dry. Season and scatter over the chilli.

Bouillabaisse

Ingredients

1 leek, green top left whole, white finely sliced

small bunch fresh thyme

3 bay leaves

bunch parsley, stalks whole, leaves roughly chopped

2 strips of orange peel

1 mild red chilli

4 tbsp olive oil

2 onions, chopped

1 leek

1 fennel, fronds picked and reserved, fennel chopped

4 garlic cloves, minced

1 tbsp tomato purée

1 star anise

2 tbsp Pernod, optional, if you have it

4 large, ripe tomatoes, chopped

large pinch (⅓ tsp) saffron strands

1 ½l fish stock

100g potato, one peeled piece

1kg of filleted mixed Mediterranean fish, each fillet cut into large chunks. (We used a mix of red and grey mullet, monkfish, John Dory and gurnard)

300g mussels, optional

For the rouille

2 garlic cloves

1 small chunk of red chilli (optional)

small pinch saffron

1 piece of potato, cooked in the broth, (see above)

1 egg yolk

100ml olive oil

1 tbsp lemon juice

For the croutons

½ baguette, thinly sliced

1 tbsp olive oil

Directions

STEP 1

To make the croutons heat oven to 200C/180C fan/gas 6. Lay the slices of bread on a flat baking tray in a single layer, drizzle with olive oil and bake for 15 mins until golden and crisp. Set aside – can be made a day ahead and kept in an airtight container.

STEP 2

Use a layer of the green part of the leek to wrap around and make a herb bundle with the thyme, bay, parsley stalks, orange peel and chilli. Tie everything together with kitchen string and set aside.

STEP 3

Heat the oil in a very large casserole dish or stock pot and throw in the onion, sliced leek and fennel and cook for about 10 mins until softened. Stir through the garlic and cook for 2 mins more, then add the herb bundle, tomato purée, star anise, Pernod if using, chopped tomatoes and saffron. Simmer and stir for a minute or two then pour over the fish stock. Season with salt and pepper, bring to a simmer, then add the piece of potato. Bubble everything gently for 30 mins until you have a thin tomatoey soup. When that piece of potato is on the brink of collapse, fish it out and set aside to make the rouille.

STEP 4

While the broth is simmering make the rouille by crushing the garlic, chilli and saffron with a pinch of salt in a mortar with a pestle. Mash in the cooked potato to make a sticky paste then whisk in the egg yolk and, very gradually, the olive oil until you make a mayonnaise-like sauce. Stir in the lemon juice and set aside.

STEP 5

Once the chunky tomato broth has cooked you have two options: for a rustic bouillabaisse, simply poach your fish in it along with the mussels, if you're using (just until they open) and serve. For a refined version, remove the herb bundle and star anise. Using a handheld or table-top blender, blitz the soup until smooth. Pass the soup through a sieve into a large, clean pan and bring to a gentle simmer. Starting with the densest fish, add the chunks to the broth and cook for 1 min before adding the next type. With the fish we used, the order was: monkfish, John Dory, grey mullet, snapper. When all the fish is in, scatter over the mussels, if using, and simmer everything for about 5 mins until just cooked and the mussels have opened.

STEP 6

Use a slotted spoon to carefully scoop the fish and mussels out onto a warmed serving platter, moisten with just a little broth and scatter over the chopped parsley. Bring everything to the table. Some people eat it as two courses, serving the broth with croutons and rouille first, then the fish spooned into the same bowl. Others simply serve it as a fish stew. Whichever way you choose the rouille is there to be stirred into the broth to thicken and give it a kick.

Curried cod

Ingredients

1 tbsp oil

1 onion, chopped

2 tbsp medium curry powder

thumb-sized piece ginger, peeled and finely grated

3 garlic cloves, crushed

2 x 400g cans chopped tomatoes

400g can chickpeas

4 cod fillets (about 125-150g each)

zest 1 lemon, then cut into wedges

handful coriander, roughly chopped

Directions

STEP 1

Heat the oil in a large, lidded frying pan. Cook the onion over a high heat for a few mins, then stir in the curry powder, ginger and garlic. Cook for another 1-2 mins until fragrant, then stir in the tomatoes, chickpeas and some seasoning.

STEP 2

Cook for 8-10 mins until thickened slightly, then top with the cod. Cover and cook for another 5-10 mins until the fish is cooked through. Scatter over the lemon zest and coriander, then serve with the lemon wedges to squeeze over.

Sausage, kale & gnocchi one-pot

Ingredients

1 tbsp olive oil

6 pork sausages

1 tsp chilli flakes

1 tsp fennel seeds (optional)

500g fresh gnocchi

500ml chicken stock (fresh if you can get it)

100g chopped kale

40g parmesan, finely grated

Directions

STEP 1

Heat the oil in a large high-sided frying pan over a medium heat. Squeeze the sausages straight from their skins into the pan, then use the back of a wooden spoon to break the meat up. Sprinkle in the chilli flakes and fennel seeds, if using, then fry until the sausagemeat is crisp around the edges. Remove from the pan with a slotted spoon.

STEP 2

Tip the gnocchi into the pan, fry for a minute or so, then pour in the chicken stock. Once bubbling, cover the pan with a lid and cook for 3 mins, then stir in the kale. Cook for 2 mins more or until the gnocchi is tender and the kale has wilted. Stir in the parmesan, then season with black pepper and scatter the crisp sausagemeat over the top.

DELIGHTFUL RECIPES FOR SNACK

Red curry chicken kebabs

Ingredients

2 boneless, skinless chicken breasts, cut into large chunks

2 tbsp Thai red curry paste

2 tbsp coconut milk

1 red pepper, deseeded and chopped into chunks

1 courgette, halved and cut into chunks

1 red onion, cut into large wedges

1 lime, halved, to serve

Directions

STEP 1

Fire up the barbecue or heat a griddle pan to high. Tip chicken, curry paste and coconut milk into a bowl, then mix well until the chicken is evenly coated. Thread vegetables and chicken onto skewers. Cook the skewers on the barbecue or griddle for 5-8 mins, turning every so often, until the chicken is cooked through and charred. Serve with herby rice, salad and a lime half to squeeze over.

From-the-fridge omelette

Ingredients

1 courgette

1 tbsp olive oil

4 eggs

half a teacup frozen peas (no need to defrost)

handful grated or sliced cheese (cheddar, feta, ricotta or goat's cheese work well)

Directions

STEP 1

Trim the ends off the courgette, then cut into slices about the thickness of a £1 coin. Heat the oil in your smallest non-stick frying pan (around 20cm). Tip in the courgette and cook for a couple of mins, just until it starts to turn golde. Break the eggs into a bowl and beat with a fork. Season with a little salt, if you like.

STEP 2

Add the peas to the pan, then pour in the eggs and sprinkle with the cheese. Turn the heat down really low and cook for about 10 mins until the egg has almost set. In the meantime, heat the grill to high. 3 After 10 mins on the hob, pop the pan under the hot grill for a min or two until all the egg has set. Place a cutting board or plate over the pan and flip over. Cut the omelette into wedges and serve warm, or leave to cool and serve with salad or coleslaw. Can be kept in the fridge for up to 3 days.

Banoffee s'mores

Ingredients

16 milk chocolate oat biscuits (we used Milk Chocolate Hobnobs)

8 large marshmallows (vegetarian brand, if required)

8 tsp dulce de leche

1 banana, cut into 16 slices

Directions

STEP 1

Preheat the grill to high and line a baking sheet with parchment. Put 8 Hobnobs on the tray with a marshmallow on top and grill until slightly brown and melting.

STEP 2

Put a tsp of dulce de leche on the remaining 8 Hobnobs and top with 2 banana slices. Sandwich the biscuits together.

Posh BLT

Ingredients

6 rashers smoked streaky bacon

1 tbsp maple syrup

3 tbsp mayo

½ tbsp sundried tomato paste

4 slices sourdough

6 chopped sundried tomatoes

leaves of 1 Little Gem

Directions

STEP 1

Heat the grill to high. Put the bacon on a foil-lined baking sheet and drizzle with the maple syrup. Grill for 7-10 mins until crisp. Mix the mayo with the sundried tomato paste, then spread over two of the sourdough slices. Top with the bacon, sundried tomatoes and Little Gem. Season with black pepper, top with the remaining bread and halve.

Melty ploughman's s'mores

Ingredients

16 cream crackers

8 slices of brie (about 80g) (vegetarian brand, if required)

4 tbsp pickle

Directions

STEP 1

Preheat the grill to high and line a baking sheet with parchment. Put 8 cream crackers on the baking sheet with a slice of Brie on each cracker. Grill until the cheese starts to melt.

STEP 2

Put some pickle on top and sandwich with the other cracker until the cheese oozes out the sides.

Plum & raspberry jam

Ingredients

1kg jam sugar

500g plum, stoned and roughly chopped

juice 1 lemon

500g raspberry

Directions

STEP 1

Tip the sugar into a heavy preserving pan or flameproof dish with the plums, lemon juice and half the raspberries. Heat until the sugar has dissolved, then bring to the boil and simmer for a few mins until the plums are tender. Add the rest of the raspberries to the pan.

STEP 2

Place a jam thermometer in the pan, bring to the boil, then cook over a high heat until the temperature reaches 104C. Alternatively, put a small plate in the fridge or freezer until really cold. Once the jam has been boiling for 10 mins and looks thick and syrupy, turn off the heat and pour a spoonful onto the plate. The jam is ready when it wrinkles as you push it with your finger; be careful not to burn yourself. If the jam is not ready, boil for another 3 mins, then repeat test as above, until it is ready.

STEP 3

Allow to cool for about 5 mins. Skim the surface of any scum and pack into warm sterilised jars (see tip below). Cover with wax discs and lids. Will keep in the fridge or a cold larder for up to 6 months.

Vegetable tagine with almond & chickpea couscous

Ingredients

400g pack shallot, peeled and cut in half

2 tbsp olive oil

1 large butternut squash, about 1.25kg/2 lb 12oz, peeled, deseeded and cut into bite size chunks

1 tsp ground cinnamon

½ tsp ground ginger

450ml strong-flavoured vegetable stock

12 small pitted prunes

2 tsp clear honey

2 red peppers, deseeded and cut into chunks

3 tbsp chopped coriander

2 tbsp chopped mint, plus extra for spinkling

For the couscous

250g couscous

1 tbsp harissa (Moroccan chilli paste)

400g can chickpea, rinsed and drained

handful toasted flaked almonds

Directions

STEP 1

Fry the shallots in the oil for 5 mins until they are softening and browned. Add the squash and spices, and stir for 1 min. Pour in the stock, season well, then add the prunes and honey. Cover and simmer for 8 mins.

STEP 2

Add the peppers and cook for 8-10 mins until just tender. Stir in the coriander and mint.

STEP 3

Pour 400ml boiling water over the couscous in a bowl, then stir in the harissa with ½ tsp salt. Tip in the chickpeas, then cover and leave for 5 mins. Fluff up with a fork and serve with the tagine, flaked almonds and extra mint.

6

HIGH FIBRE RECIPES YOU MUST TRY!

DELIGHTFUL RECIPES FOR BREAKFAST

High-fibre muesli

Ingredients

300g jumbo oats

100g All-Bran

25g wheatgerm

100g dark raisins

140g ready-to-eat apricots, snipped into chunks

50g golden linseed

Directions

STEP 1

Mix everything in a large bowl. You can store this for up to 2 months in an airtight container. When you're ready to serve, pour lots of chilled milk over and let it soak for a few minutes.

South American-style quinoa with fried eggs

Ingredients

75g quinoa

400g can black beans, drained

½ tsp ground cumin

½ tsp ground coriander

1 lime, zested and juiced, plus extra wedges to serve

1 tsp cider vinegar

160g cherry tomatoes, halved

1 small avocado, stoned, peeled and roughly chopped

2 tbsp finely chopped coriander

3 spring onions or ½ small red onion, finely chopped

rapeseed oil, for frying

2 medium eggs

Directions

STEP 1

Put the quinoa in a small pan with 250ml water and bring to the boil. Reduce the heat to low, cover and gently simmer for 15-20 mins, stirring occasionally until most of the water has been absorbed and the grains have doubled in size (if there's any water left in the pan, drain well).

STEP 2

Tip into a bowl and stir through the beans, spices, lime zest and juice and vinegar. Stir well, then add the tomatoes, avocado, coriander and onion, and spoon onto plates.

STEP 3

Heat a drop of oil in a non-stick frying pan and fry the eggs until the whites are set with a crispy edge and the yolk is runny. Serve the quinoa topped with the eggs.

Breakfast casserole

Ingredients

250g chestnut mushrooms, sliced

1½ tbsp vegetable oil, plus extra for the tin (optional)

6 veggie sausages, sliced into bite-sized pieces

1 large red onion, finely sliced

2 red peppers, deseeded and sliced

8 eggs

250ml whole milk

125g cheddar, grated

10g chives, finely sliced

Directions

STEP 1

Heat the oven to 200C/180C fan/gas 6. Fry the mushrooms in a large non-stick frying pan over a medium-high heat until the liquid has released and evaporated, about 8-10 mins. Add ½ tbsp oil and fry until golden, about 2 mins. Remove from the pan and tip into a large bowl.

STEP 2

Wipe out the pan to remove any excess liquid, then return to a medium heat. Add the remaining oil and fry the sausages until golden all over. Remove using a slotted spoon and add to the bowl with the mushrooms. Fry the onions and peppers, stirring occasionally for 8-10 mins until soft but not browned. Tip into the bowl with the sausages and mushrooms, and mix everything together to combine. Season well. Tip the sausage and veg mixture into a baking dish (around 35 x 25cm) or roasting tin. If you're using a tin, you may need to oil it to prevent the casserole from sticking.

STEP 3

Combine the eggs, milk, cheddar and chives in a large jug, season well, then pour this over the Ingredients in the dish or tin. Bake for 25-30 mins until golden and set. Leave to cool slightly before cutting into squares.

Slow cooker bio yogurt

Ingredients

2l whole milk

100ml live yogurt, either shop bought or from a previous homemade batch

Directions

STEP 1

Tip the milk into the slow cooker. Cover and heat on High until the temperature of the milk reaches 82C, this will take a couple of hours. Turn off the slow cooker and allow the temperature to drop to 43C for a further 2-3 hours. Take a mugful of the warm milk and mix it with the yogurt then pour the mixture back into the slow cooker and stir really well. Cover, wrap the slow cooker in a big towel and then leave undisturbed for 9-12 hours until the mixture has set.

STEP 2

Eat on top of cereal or porridge, topped with fresh fruit, in marinades or drink in smoothies. If you want it thicker, for dips for example, line a large sieve with muslin and place it over a bowl, tip in the yogurt and allow some of the whey to strain off until you get the consistency of yogurt that you like. The longer you leave it, the thicker it will become. Store in the fridge for up to 2 weeks.

Staffordshire oatcakes with mushrooms

Ingredients

For the oatcakes

85g porridge oats

85g plain wholemeal flour

½ tsp dried yeast

For the topping

4 tsp rapeseed oil, plus a little for frying

320g button mushrooms, sliced

4 tomatoes, each cut into 8 wedges

4 tbsp milled seeds with flax and chia

4 tbsp tahini

a few coriander sprigs, chopped

Directions

STEP 1

For the oatcakes, tip the oats and 350ml water into a bowl and blitz with a stick blender until smooth (alternatively you can use a food processor or liquidizer). Stir in the flour and yeast, cover and leave in the fridge overnight, or leave at room temperature for 2-3 hrs until bubbles appear.

STEP 2

Use kitchen paper to rub ½ tsp oil round a non-stick frying pan, then heat. Ladle in a quarter of the batter and swirl the pan to cover the base (the oatcakes should be a few millimeters thick, like a crêpe). Cook for 2 mins, then turn and cook for 2 mins more until golden. Make four oatcakes in the same way. If you're following our Healthy Diet Plan, chill two for another day. Will keep, covered in the fridge, for two days.

STEP 3

To make the topping for two oatcakes, heat 2 tsp oil in a non-stick pan, add 160g mushrooms and fry for

2-3 mins, stirring until softened. Stir in 2 tomatoes, then add 2 tbsp ground seeds and cook for 2 mins more. Reheat the oatcakes in a dry frying pan or the microwave if necessary, then spread each one with 1 tbsp tahini, the mushroom mixture and scatter with a little coriander before serving. On the second day, repeat step 3 with the remaining Ingredients.

Sweetcorn pancakes

Ingredients

a whole corn on the cob or a 330g can of sweetcorn, drained

2medium eggs

5 tbsp milk

25g butter, melted

85g self-raising flour

2 spring onions, finely chopped

4 tbsp sunflower oil, for shallow frying

To serve

4 tomatoes, cut in half

olive oil, for drizzling

8rashers good quality bacon, streaky or back

chilli sauce to serve

Directions

STEP 1

First turn the grill on high. If using fresh corn,
remove the husk and slice the kernels from the cob
with a large sharp knife, then cook them in a pan of

boiling water for 5 minutes. Drain and leave to cool while you whisk the eggs, milk and butter together. Whisk in the flour and a large pinch of salt until smooth, then mix in the corn (fresh or canned) and the spring onions.

STEP 2

Put the tomatoes cut-side up on a large baking tray, drizzle with olive oil and season with salt and pepper. Lay the bacon next to the tomatoes in a single file on the tray. Grill for 8–10 minutes until the tomatoes have softened and the bacon is crispy, turning the rashers over at half time.

STEP 3

While the bacon's crisping up, heat the sunflower oil in a large frying pan. Add 4 large spoonfuls of the batter and fry for 1-2 minutes on each side until the pancakes are puffed up and golden. Lift out on to a plate lined with kitchen paper and cook the remaining 4 pancakes. Bring to the table with a bottle of chilli sauce.

Banana overnight oats

Ingredients

2 bananas, peeled

100g porridge oats

¼ tsp ground cinnamon, plus a pinch to serve

1 tbsp maple syrup

300ml milk of your choice, plus a splash

2 tbsp peanut or almond butter, plus extra to serve

2 tbsp flaked or chopped almonds

2-4 tbsp natural yogurt, to serve (optional)

Directions

STEP 1

Mash 1 banana in a bowl with a fork until smooth. Stir in the oats, cinnamon, maple syrup, milk and peanut butter. Mix well, then cover and chill overnight.

STEP 2

The next morning, stir the porridge, adding another splash of milk if the mixture is quite stiff. Divide between two bowls. Slice the remaining banana and scatter this over the porridge, drizzle with more nut butter and sprinkle over the almonds. Top with spoonfuls of yogurt, if using, and sprinkle with a pinch more cinnamon before serving.

DELIGHTFUL RECIPES FOR LUNCH

Spinach & tomato tortillas

Ingredients

1 tsp olive oil

1 onion, chopped

1 red or yellow pepper, seeded and chopped

200g can chopped tomato

85g canned mixed bean, rinsed and drained

good pinch of mild chilli powder

3generous handfuls of fresh spinach leaves

4 flour tortillas, about 20cm in diameter

Directions

STEP 1

Heat the olive oil in a frying pan, add the onion and pepper and cook gently for a few minutes until they are soft.

STEP 2

Tip in the tomatoes and mixed beans, then add the chilli powder. Heat until the sauce is bubbling, then lower the heat and simmer gently for 10 minutes. Now add the spinach to the tomato and bean mixture and cook until the leaves have wilted – this will only take a minute or so. Remove the pan from the heat. Check the seasoning – you shouldn't need salt, though you might want to add a little pepper, and more chilli powder if you like things hot.

Harissa vegetables with quinoa

Ingredients

1 tbsp rapeseed oil

2 red onions (160g), chopped

1 green pepper, deseeded and cubed

1 small sweet potato (200g), peeled and cut into chunks

2 large celery sticks (125g), cut into chunky slices

10g ginger, finely chopped

300ml vegetable stock made with 2 tsp vegan bouillon powder

1 tbsp harissa paste

2 tbsp tomato purée

2 dried apricots, quartered

10g coriander or parsley, chopped, plus a few extra leaves to serve

250g pack cooked red and white quinoa

4 tbsp coconut yogurt

Directions

STEP 1

Heat the oil in a non-stick pan and fry the vegetables and ginger for 10 mins, stirring frequently, until softened and starting to colour.

STEP 2

Stir in the stock, harissa, tomato purée and apricots. Bring to the boil, cover and simmer for 15 mins. Stir in the coriander.

STEP 3

Meanwhile, heat the quinoa following pack instructions. Serve with the veg and yogurt, plus a scattering of coriander leaves.

Courgette, chilli & mint with pearl couscous

Ingredients

100g pearl couscous

1 tbsp olive oil

400g courgettes, roughly chopped

½ red onion, sliced

1 red chilli (deseeded if you prefer less heat), finely chopped

2 garlic cloves, finely sliced

10g mint, leaves picked and finely chopped, plus a few whole to serve

½ lemon, juiced

1 tbsp honey

50g light Greek-style salad cheese

Directions

STEP 1

Cook the couscous following pack instructions, then drain and set aside. Meanwhile, heat the oil in a frying pan over a medium-high heat. Tip in the courgettes and onion and fry, stirring occasionally, until browned and softened, about 8-10 mins. Stir in the chilli and garlic and cook for a further 2-3 mins until fragrant.

STEP 2

Remove from the heat and stir through the chopped mint, lemon juice, honey and seasoning. Divide the couscous between plates, top with the courgette mix, crumble over the cheese and scatter with the whole mint leaves to serve.

Tuna, spring onion & sweetcorn fritters

Ingredients

125ml milk

3 eggs, beaten

150g self-raising flour

300g frozen sweetcorn, defrosted (or use cooked fresh corn)

½ bunch of spring onions, trimmed and thinly sliced

1 lemon, zested and cut into wedges

2 x 112g cans tuna, drained and roughly flaked

sunflower or vegetable oil, for frying

To serve

100g soured cream

hot sauce, to serve (optional)

Directions

STEP 1

Mix the milk and eggs together in a jug with ½ tsp salt and ¼ tsp ground black pepper. Sift the flour into a bowl, make a well in the centre and pour in the egg mixture in a thin, steady stream, whisking well until combined. Stir in the sweetcorn, spring onions, lemon zest and tuna.

STEP 2

Heat a drop of oil in a non-stick or cast iron frying pan over a medium heat. Drop spoonfuls of the batter into the pan and cook until crisp and golden, about 2-3 mins, flip and repeat on the other side (you'll need to do this in batches). Keep warm in a low oven and repeat with the remaining batter.

Spiced lentil & butternut squash soup

Ingredients

2 tbsp olive oil

2 onions, finely chopped

2 garlic cloves, crushed

¼ tsp hot chilli powder

1 tbsp ras el hanout

1 butternut squash, peeled and cut into 2cm pieces

100g red lentils

1l hot vegetable stock

1 small bunch coriander, leaves chopped, plus extra to serve

dukkah (see tip) and natural yogurt, to serve

Directions

STEP 1

Heat the oil in a large flameproof casserole dish or saucepan over a medium-high heat. Fry the onions with a pinch of salt for 7 mins, or until softened and just caramelised. Add the garlic, chilli and ras el hanout, and cook for 1 min more.

STEP 2

Stir in the squash and lentils. Pour over the stock and season to taste. Bring to the boil, then reduce the heat to a simmer and cook, covered, for 25 mins or until the squash is soft. Blitz the soup with a stick blender until smooth, then season to taste. To freeze, leave to cool completely and transfer to large freezerproof bags.

STEP 3

Stir in the coriander leaves and ladle the soup into bowls. Serve topped with the dukkah, yogurt and extra coriander leaves.

Leek & broccoli soup with cheesy scones

Ingredients

375g leeks, thinly sliced

400g potatoes, peeled and cut into medium chunks

2 garlic cloves, chopped

2 tsp vegetable bouillon powder

340g broccoli, roughly chopped

250ml milk

For the cheese scones

165g plain wholemeal flour

1 tsp baking powder

20g parmesan or vegetarian alternative, finely grated

1 tsp mustard powder

100ml milk

½ tbsp olive oil

65g soft goat's cheese

4 tomatoes, sliced, to serve

Directions

STEP 1

Tip the leeks, potatoes and garlic into a large pan with the bouillon. Pour over 800ml boiling water, stir well, cover and simmer for 15 mins.

STEP 2

Add the broccoli to the pan, then cover and cook for 5 mins more until just tender. Blitz with a hand blender until smooth, then pour in the milk and blitz again. Add a little stock if the soup looks too thick.

STEP 3

To make the scones, heat the oven to 220C/200C fan/gas 7 and line a baking tray with baking parchment. Put the flour and baking powder in a bowl with the all but 1 tbsp of the parmesan and all the mustard powder. Gradually add the milk and oil, stirring with a cutlery knife until the mixture comes together. Shape into a log, about 16cm long and 6cm wide, and press the remaining parmesan on top. Cut in half along the length, then halve each of those pieces again to create four wedge-like scones. Arrange the scones on the tray and bake for 10-12 mins until golden.

Curried bean & coconut cod

Ingredients

125g brown basmati rice

200g can sweetcorn

15g ginger, peeled

2 large garlic cloves

½ tsp mustard seeds

1 tbsp garam masala

1 tsp vegetable bouillon powder

½-1 red chilli, deseeded and sliced (optional)

1 cinnamon stick

160g green beans, trimmed

160g whole cherry tomatoes

160g baby spinach

2 skinless cod loins (about 240g)

80g coconut yogurt

10g coriander, chopped, plus extra to serve

Directions

STEP 1

Boil the rice following pack instructions. Meanwhile, tip the sweetcorn into a bowl with the ginger and garlic, and blitz with a hand blender until smooth and creamy.

STEP 2

Put the mustard seeds in a large pan and warm briefly over a low heat until they start to pop. Tip in the garam masala and sweetcorn mixture, and mix with 350ml boiling water, the bouillon, chilli (if using) and cinnamon stick. Bring to the boil, then lower the heat to medium. Add the beans and tomatoes, then cover the pan and cook for 6 mins.

STEP 3

Add the spinach and stir until beginning to wilt, then top with the fish, spoon over some sauce or gently push it under, then cover and cook 5-8 mins more until the fish is just cooked.

STEP 4

Carefully lift the fish from the pan and stir the coconut yogurt and coriander into the curry. Serve with the rice and extra coriander scattered over.

DELIGHTFUL RECIPES FOR DINNER

Red lentil & squash dhal

Ingredients

1 tbsp sunflower oil

1 onion, finely chopped

1 garlic clove, finely chopped

1 tsp ground coriander

1 tsp ground cumin

1 tsp ground turmeric

½ tsp cayenne pepper

400g butternut squash, peeled and cut into 2cm (prepared weight)

400g can chopped tomato

1.2l chicken stock

1 heaped tbsp mango chutney

300g red lentil

small pack coriander, roughly chopped

naan bread, to serve

Directions

STEP 1

Put the oil and the onion in a saucepan, and cook for 5 mins. Stir in the garlic and cook for a further 1 min, then stir in the spices and butternut squash. Combine everything together.

STEP 2

Tip in the chopped tomatoes, stock and chutney, and season well. Bring to the boil, then gently simmer for about 10 mins. Add the lentils and simmer for another 20 mins until the lentils and squash are tender. Stir in the coriander and serve with warmed naan bread.

Squid, prawn & chickpea nduja stew

Ingredients

2 tbsp olive oil

1 onion, finely chopped

1 fennel, finely chopped, fronds reserved

2 garlic cloves, sliced

1 tbsp nduja or 1 cooking chorizo, skin removed, crumbled

400g can chopped tomatoes

100ml red wine

250ml chicken stock

400g can chickpeas, drained

200g prepared squid

200g king prawns (peeled weight)

small handful of flat-leaf parsley, chopped

1 lemon, zested

Directions

STEP 1

Heat the olive oil in a large, flameproof shallow casserole dish over a medium heat, and cook the onion, fennel and garlic for 12 mins, stirring occasionally until soft and just turning golden. Stir in the nduja or chorizo and sizzle for 2 mins until the oils are released and the veg starts to take on the red colour.

STEP 2

Tip in the tomatoes, then rinse the can out with the wine and pour it in, along with the stock. Stir in the chickpeas. Season and bring to a simmer, then cook for 20 mins until the sauce is rich. Season to taste.

STEP 3

Stir in the squid and prawns so they're completely mixed into the sauce, then simmer for about 5 mins more until the squid and prawns are cooked through. Scatter with the parsley, lemon zest and reserved fennel fronds before serving.

Curried satay noodles

Ingredients

150g dried wholewheat noodles

2 tsp rapeseed oil

1 red pepper, halved seeded and thinly sliced

1 carrot, cut into matchsticks (about 90g)

1 tbsp finely chopped ginger

3 garlic cloves, finely chopped

1 chilli, deseeded and finely chopped (optional)

½ tsp cumin seeds

1-2 tsp curry powder

2 ½ -3 tbsp crunchy peanut butter

1 tbsp tomato purée

150ml vegetable stock, made with ½ tsp vegetable bouillon

100g frozen peas

½ lemon, juiced

Directions

STEP 1

Boil the noodles following pack instructions, then rinse well to ensure the strands are separate. Meanwhile, heat the oil in a wok or sauté pan over a high heat and stir-fry the pepper, carrot, ginger, garlic and chilli, if using, for 5 mins until softened.

Stir in the cumin seeds and curry powder and cook for 30 seconds or so until aromatic.

STEP 2

Mix the peanut butter and tomato purée with the vegetable stock until smooth. Add the drained noodles to the wok along with the frozen peas, then pour in the peanut and tomato mixture and toss everything together. If it seems a bit claggy, stir in a drop more water. Squeeze in the lemon juice, toss well and serve.

Smoky chickpeas on toast

Ingredients

1 tsp olive oil or vegetable oil, plus a drizzle

1 small onion or banana shallot, chopped

2 tsp chipotle paste

250ml passata

400g can chickpeas, drained

2 tsp honey

2 tsp red wine vinegar

2-4 slices good crusty bread

2 eggs

Directions

STEP 1

Heat ½ tsp of the oil in a pan. Tip in the onion and cook until soft, about 5-8 mins, then add the chipotle paste, passata, chickpeas, honey and vinegar. Season and bubble for 5 mins.

STEP 2

Toast the bread. Heat the remaining oil in a frying pan and fry the eggs. Drizzle the toast with a little oil, then top with the chickpeas and fried eggs.

Posh egg, chips & beans

Ingredients

4 large baking potatoes, cut into wedges

2 tbsp olive oil

1 onion, finely chopped

1 tsp smoked paprika

1 thyme sprig

400g can chopped tomatoes

2 x 400g cans cannellini beans

4 eggs

handful chopped flat-leaf parsley

Directions

STEP 1

Heat oven to 200C/180C fan/gas 6. Tip the potatoes into a large roasting tin and toss with 1 tbsp of the oil and some seasoning. Bake for 45 mins-1 hr until crisp and golden, tossing them again halfway through.

STEP 2

Meanwhile, heat the remaining oil in a pan. Add the onion and cook for 10-15 mins until starting to soften, then add the paprika, thyme, chopped tomatoes and beans (including the liquid from the can) and stir well. Simmer for 15 mins, or until thickened, then discard the thyme sprig.

STEP 3

Fry or poach the eggs. Serve alongside the wedges and beans and garnish with the parsley.

Lentil & tuna salad

Ingredients

2 tbsp sherry vinegar

1 tsp Dijon mustard

2 garlic cloves, finely grated

50ml olive oil

2 x 250g pouches ready-cooked puy lentils

2 x 160g cans tuna steaks in spring water, drained and flaked

160g cherry tomatoes, halved (about 10)

2 ready-roasted peppers, chopped

handful of parsley, finely chopped

½ small bunch of chives, finely chopped, plus extra to garnish

Directions

STEP 1

Whisk the vinegar, mustard and garlic together in a small bowl. Slowly drizzle in the oil, whisking as you go, until emulsified, then season to taste.

STEP 2

Add the lentils, tuna, tomatoes, peppers and herbs to a large bowl and toss together. Pour over the dressing and toss again. Divide between four bowls and garnish with the remaining chives.

Roasted carrot & whipped feta tart

Ingredients

large bunch of carrots with tops (about 800g)

2 tsp olive oil

1 tsp za'atar

2 tsp honey

125-150ml extra virgin olive oil

2 garlic cloves, roughly chopped

50g walnuts, roughly chopped

40g grated parmesan or vegetarian hard cheese

25g parsley, roughly chopped, plus whole leaves to serve

200g feta drained and crumbled (vegetarian, if needed)

150g Greek yogurt

1 lemon, zested

500g block puff pastry

1 egg, beaten

Directions

STEP 1

Heat the oven to 200C/180C fan/gas 6. Trim off the carrot tops, discarding any tough stems, then set aside. Halve the carrots lengthways, tip into a roasting tin and toss with the olive oil and some seasoning. Roast for 25-30 mins until tender and golden, stirring once or twice to ensure they don't stick. Stir in the za'atar and honey, and set aside.

STEP 2

Meanwhile, tip the reserved carrot tops and extra virgin olive oil into a food processor. Season and blitz, scraping down the sides occasionally until finely chopped. Add the garlic, walnuts, parmesan and parsley, and pulse until combined. Pour in another splash of olive oil, if needed. Transfer to a bowl and season to taste. Clean out the food processor, then tip in the feta, yogurt, most of the lemon zest and some seasoning. Blitz until smooth and creamy.

STEP 3

Put a large baking tray in the oven to heat up. Roll the pastry out on a sheet of baking parchment into a roughly 40 x 30cm rectangle. Gently score a 2cm border around the edge using a sharp knife. Brush the beaten egg all over the pastry and sprinkle a large pinch of sea salt around the border. Carefully slide the pastry onto the hot baking tray using the parchment to help you, and bake for 15-20 mins until golden and puffed up. Remove from the oven and gently press the middle down using the back of a metal spoon. Cool for 5-10 mins, then spread the whipped feta over the middle and arrange the roasted carrots on top. Drizzle over the pesto, scatter over the parsley and the remaining lemon zest, and cut into slices to serve.

DELIGHTFUL RECIPES FOR SNACK

Aubergine couscous salad

Ingredients

1 large aubergine, sliced into 1cm rounds

3 tbsp olive oil

140g couscous

225ml hot vegetable stock

200g cherry tomato, halved

handful mint leaves, roughly chopped

100g log firm goat's cheese, cubed

juice ½ lemon

Instructions

STEP 1

Heat grill to high. Put the aubergine on a baking sheet, brush with oil and season. Grill for about 15 mins, turning and brushing with more oil halfway, until browned and softened.

STEP 2

Meanwhile, tip the couscous into a large bowl, pour over the stock, then cover and leave for 10 mins. Mix the tomatoes, mint, goat's cheese and remaining oil together. Fluff the couscous up with a fork, then stir in the aubergines, tomato mixture and lemon juice.

Spanish spinach omelette

Ingredients

400g bag spinach leaves

3 tbsp olive oil

1 large onion, finely sliced

2 large potatoes, peeled and finely sliced

10 eggs

Instructions

STEP 1

Tip the spinach into a large colander and bring a kettleful of water to the boil. Slowly pour the water over the spinach until wilted, then cool under cold water. Squeeze all the liquid out of the spinach and set aside.

STEP 2

Heat grill to high. Heat the oil in a non-stick frying pan and gently cook the onion and potato for about 10 mins until the potato is soft. While the onion is cooking, beat the eggs together in a large bowl and season with salt and pepper. Stir the spinach into the potatoes, then pour in the eggs and cook, stirring occasionally, until nearly set, then flash the omelette under the grill to set the top. Ease the omelette on to a plate, then flip over back into the pan. Finish cooking the omelette on the underside and turn out onto a board. Serve cut into wedges.

Chicken & orange salad

Ingredients

150g pack green bean, trimmed

1 fennel bulb

1 large avocado

100g bag watercress, roughly chopped

2 oranges

2 tbsp olive oil

2 cooked chicken breasts, shredded

Instructions

STEP 1

Cook the beans in a large pan of boiling salted water
for 4-5 mins. Cool under cold water and put in a
bowl. Finely slice the fennel bulb, cutting away the
core.

STEP 2

Peel and slice the avocado and add to bowl with
watercress. Peel the oranges, cut out the segments

and add to bowl. Squeeze the rest of the orange juice into a bowl and mix with the olive oil to make a dressing. Toss salad in the dressing, scatter over chicken, then serve.

Spinach baked eggs with parmesan & tomato toasts

Ingredients

400g fresh spinach

100g Basil, parmesan (or vegetarian alternative) & tomato butter

4 eggs

8-12 slices French stick

Instructions

STEP 1

Heat oven to 190C/fan 170C/gas 5. Wash the spinach and trim off any thick stalks. Put into a large pan, then cook, covered, until the spinach is wilted, about 2-3 mins. Drain well, pressing out all excess water, then return to the pan with about a quarter of the butter, stirring until the spinach is glistening.

STEP 2

Heat grill to high. Divide the spinach between 4 buttered ramekins, then break an egg into each. Season with salt and pepper, then top with a slice of butter. Bake for 10-12 mins, until the eggs are just set. Meanwhile, grill the bread on one side until crisp, then spread the untoasted side with the remaining butter and grill again until crisp. Serve the eggs with the toast on the side.

Brummie bacon cakes

Ingredients

3 rashers streaky bacon (we used smoked)

225g self-raising flour, plus extra for dusting

25g butter, cold and cut into small pieces

75g mature cheddar, grated

150ml milk, plus 2 tbsp extra for glazing

1 tbsp tomato ketchup

½ tsp Worcestershire sauce

Instructions

STEP 1

Heat grill to high and grill the bacon for 10 mins, turning halfway, until crisp. Cool for a few mins. Meanwhile, heat oven to 180C/160C fan/gas 4 and line a baking sheet with parchment. Sift the flour and ½ tsp salt into a bowl, add the butter, then rub in to the texture of fine breadcrumbs. Cut the bacon into small pieces and add to the bowl with a third of the cheese.

STEP 2

Mix the milk, ketchup and Worcestershire sauce in a jug. Pour into the bacon mixture, stirring briefly, to make a soft dough. Flour the work surface, turn the dough onto it and shape into an 18cm round. Brush with milk, then cut into 8 wedges with a large knife.

STEP 3

Arrange the wedges on the baking sheet and sprinkle with the remaining cheese. Bake for 20-30 mins or until risen and golden brown, and serve warm (or cool on a wire rack, and store in an airtight container). Warm the bacon cakes through in a low oven (140C/120C fan/gas 1) if you've made them in advance.

Microwave butternut squash risotto

Ingredients

250g risotto rice

700ml hot vegetable stock

1 medium butternut squash

big handful grated parmesan (or vegetarian alternative), plus extra handful sage leaves, roughly chopped

Instructions

STEP 1

Tip the rice into a large bowl, then add 500ml of the hot vegetable stock. Cover with cling film and microwave on High for 5 mins. Meanwhile, peel and cut the squash into medium chunks (see tip, below). Stir the rice, then add the squash and the rest of the stock. Re-cover with cling film, then microwave for another 15 mins, stirring halfway, until almost all the stock is absorbed and the rice and squash are tender.

STEP 2

Leave the risotto to sit for 2 mins, then stir in the parmesan and sage. Serve topped with more grated cheese.

Burmese tofu fritters (tohu jaw)

Ingredients

2 tbsp vegetable oil, plus extra for the dish and fryer

100g gram flour

¼ tsp salt

1 tsp vegetable bouillon powder

¼ tsp ground turmeric

¼ tsp baking powder

For the dipping sauce

1 ½ tbsp golden caster sugar

2 tbsp fish sauce

2 tbsp light soy sauce

2 limes, juiced

2 finger chillies, sliced into rings

3 garlic cloves, crushed

Instructions

STEP 1

Mix all the Ingredients for the dipping sauce in a bowl. Cover and set aside.

STEP 2

Oil a 15 x 20cm casserole dish. Put the flour, salt, bouillon powder, turmeric, baking powder and 350ml water in a large bowl and whisk thoroughly. Cover and leave somewhere cool for 2 hrs, whisking occasionally.

STEP 3

Pour 250ml boiling water into a large saucepan over a high heat. Add the oil, then pour in the flour mixture and stir slowly with a large spoon. Reduce the heat to medium-high. Continue stirring for up to 10 mins until the mixture starts to bubble and forms a thick, custard-like consistency. Pour into the casserole dish and leave at room temperature to set and cool completely.

STEP 4

Drain away any excess liquid, wrap the tofu in kitchen paper and place back in the dish. At this point, you can cover and chill for up to 48 hrs until needed.

STEP 5

When you're ready to fry the fritters, unwrap the tofu and slice it into 5 x 3 x 1cm rectangles.

STEP 6

Heat a wok or deep-fat fryer with 5cm of oil (no more than one-third full) until you can feel waves of heat when you hold your hand 10cm above the fryer. Gently lower 3 or 4 tofu rectangles into the hot oil – they should start to sizzle almost at once. Fry for 3 mins until golden, then flip gently and fry for a further 3 mins. Remove with a slotted spoon and drain in a colander set over a dish to catch excess oil. Repeat with the next batch.

STEP 7

When you've fried all the tofu fritters, tip them back into the hot oil and fry for a further 4-5 mins for extra crispness. Drain the tofu fritters on plenty of kitchen paper and serve with the garlic dipping sauce or a sweet chilli sauce.

7

LOW CALORIES RECIPES YOU MUST TRY!

DELIGHTFUL RECIPES FOR BREAKFAST

Norwegian custard buns

Ingredients

50g unsalted butter

350ml milk

475g plain flour

100g caster sugar

7g sachet fast-action dried yeast

1½ tsp ground cardamom

1 egg, beaten

50g icing sugar

50g desiccated coconut

For the custard

250ml milk

100ml double cream

1 tsp vanilla extract

2 egg yolks (freeze the whites to use in another recipe)

50g caster sugar

2 tbsp cornflour

Instructions

STEP 1

Warm the butter and milk together in a pan over a low heat until the butter has melted. Remove from the heat and leave to cool for a few minutes until just tepid. Meanwhile, tip the flour, sugar, yeast, cardamom and ½ tsp salt into the bowl of a stand mixer fitted with a dough hook. Pour the warm milk and butter mixture into the dry Ingredients and stir to combine, then knead for 5 mins until you have a smooth dough. Or, knead by hand in a large bowl for 8-10 mins. Cover and leave to prove in a warm place until the dough has doubled in size, about 1 hr 30 mins.

STEP 2

For the custard, warm the milk, cream and vanilla in a pan over a low heat until beginning to steam.

Whisk the egg yolks, sugar and cornflour together in a large heatproof bowl, then gradually pour in the hot milk mixture, whisking continuously. Pour the mixture back into the pan and heat gently, stirring occasionally for 5-6 mins until thickened into a custard. Pour into a heatproof bowl, cover with a circle of baking parchment and leave to cool, then chill until ready to use.

STEP 3

Line one or two baking trays with baking parchment. Knock the dough back, then divide into 12 pieces (about 70g each) and form into smooth balls. Arrange over the trays, spacing well apart, then cover and leave to prove for 30 mins.

STEP 4

Heat the oven to 200C/180C fan/gas 6. Make a gap in the centre of each dough ball, roughly the size of an egg yolk. Spoon the chilled custard into each gap, then brush the exposed dough with the beaten egg. Bake for 18-22 mins until golden and risen. Leave to cool completely.

STEP 5

Mix the icing sugar with 2 tsp water, then brush over the exposed dough. Sprinkle with the desiccated coconut and leave to set slightly before serving.

Slow cooker breakfast beans

Ingredients

1 tbsp olive oil

1 onion, thinly sliced

2 garlic cloves, chopped

1 tbsp white or red wine vinegar

1 heaped tbsp soft brown sugar

400g can pinto beans, drained and rinsed

200ml passata

small bunch coriander, chopped

Instructions

STEP 1

Heat the slow cooker if necessary. Heat the oil in a large frying pan and fry the onion until it starts to brown, then add the garlic and cook for 1 min. Add the vinegar and sugar and bubble for a minute. Stir in the beans and passata and season with black pepper. Tip everything into the slow cooker.

STEP 2

Cook on Low for 5 hours. If the sauce seems a little thin turn the heat to High and cook for a few more minutes. Stir through the coriander.

Millet porridge with almond milk & berry compote

Ingredients

340g millet

1 litre unsweetened fortified almond milk, plus extra to serve

few mint leaves, to serve

For the compote

90g pitted dates, finely chopped

500g frozen mixed fruit (ours was a mixed bag of berries, cherries, currants and strawberries)

1 cinnamon stick

Instructions

STEP 1

For the compote, put the dates in a pan with 150ml water, bring to the boil and stir well so they break down. Tip in the frozen fruit and cinnamon stick and cook over a medium heat, stirring every now and then for a couple of minutes. Don't worry about fully thawing larger fruits, as they will defrost in the residual heat and retain their shape in the compote (if you have large strawberries in the mix, you can halve these as they soften). Leave to cool. Will then keep chilled for up to four days.

STEP 2

Rinse the millet in a sieve, then tip into a deep, heavy-based saucepan and pour in the almond milk and 350ml water. Put over a low heat and once bubbling, leave to simmer for 10-12 mins, stirring frequently until the millet grains are tender, but nutty.

STEP 3

Serve a third of the porridge with a third of the compote, between two people, on the first day of the Healthy Diet Plan. Add a little extra almond milk to serve with a few mint leaves scattered over. Chill the remainder for the subsequent two days. Will keep covered and chilled for up to four days. To serve on another day, reheat portions of the porridge in a pan with extra almond milk or water to loosen. Serve with the chilled compote.

Panettone French toast

Ingredients

3 eggs

150ml whole milk

1 tsp mixed spice

2 tbsp double cream

3 tbsp brandy

40g unsalted butter

4 tbsp mixed dried fruit

4 slices panettone (around 320g), cut in half to make 8

60g crème fraîche, to serve

maple syrup, to serve (optional)

2 tsp icing sugar, to serve

Instructions

STEP 1

Tip the eggs, milk, mixed spice, double cream and 1 tbsp brandy into a jug and beat to combine, then pour the mixture into a large, shallow dish.

STEP 2

Pour the remaining brandy into a cold frying pan along with 15g butter and the mixed fruit. Warm over a low heat for 3-4 mins until the butter has melted and the liquid has thickened slightly. Pour the fruit mixture into a small heatproof bowl and set aside.

STEP 3

Lay the panettone slices in the egg mixture and flip over to soak. Do this quickly so it doesn't break apart. Set aside on a plate.

STEP 4

Melt the remaining butter over a medium-low heat in the frying pan you used earlier, and fry the panettone slices for 3-4 mins on each side until golden and cooked through. It's easier to do this over a lower heat so the outside doesn't burn before the centre cooks.

STEP 5

Divide the slices between four plates, then top with the crème fraîche, mixed fruit, a little maple syrup (if using) and a dusting of icing sugar.

Chia & oat breakfast bowl

Ingredients

100g frozen raspberries

1 orange, ½ sliced, ½ juiced

150g porridge oats

100ml milk

2 tbsp smooth almond butter

½ banana, peeled and sliced

1 tbsp goji berries

1 tbsp chia seeds

Instructions

STEP 1

Tip half the raspberries and all of the orange juice into a pan. Simmer until the raspberries soften, about 5 mins.

STEP 2

Meanwhile, stir the oats, milk and 450ml water together in a pan over a low heat until creamy. Serve topped with the raspberry compote, almond butter, remaining raspberries, orange slices, banana slices, goji berries and chia seeds.

Homemade granola

Ingredients

2 tbsp vegetable oil

125ml maple syrup

2 tbsp honey

1 tsp vanilla extract

300g rolled oats

50g sunflower seed

4 tbsp sesame seeds

50g pumpkin seeds

100g flaked almond

100g dried berries (find them in the baking aisle)

50g coconut flakes or desiccated coconut

Instructions

STEP 1

Heat oven to 150C/fan 130C/gas 2. Mix the oil, maple syrup, honey and vanilla in a large bowl. Tip in all the remaining Ingredients, except the dried fruit and coconut, and mix well.

STEP 2

Tip the granola onto two baking sheets and spread evenly. Bake for 15 mins, then mix in the coconut and dried fruit, and bake for 10-15 mins more. Remove and scrape onto a flat tray to cool. Serve with cold milk or yogurt. The granola can be stored in an airtight container for up to a month.

Leftover porridge pancakes

Ingredients

150g cold leftover porridge

150g self-raising flour

2 tsp baking powder

1 ripe banana, mashed

2 large eggs

100ml milk

2 tsp vegetable or sunflower oil

fruit, yogurt and maple syrup or honey, to serve

Instructions

STEP 1

Mix the porridge, flour, baking powder, banana, eggs and milk in a bowl. Heat the oil in a frying pan. Drop 2-3 tbsp of the porridge mixture into the pan and cook over a medium heat until the underside is golden and bubbles are popping on the surface.

STEP 2

Flip over and cook for another few mins until cooked through, then keep warm in a low oven and repeat until you've used up all the batter. Serve with the fruit and yogurt and top with a drizzle of the syrup or honey.

Miso mushroom & tofu noodle soup

Ingredients

1 tbsp rapeseed oil

70g mixed mushrooms, sliced

50g smoked tofu, cut into small cubes

½ tbsp brown rice miso paste

50g dried buckwheat or egg noodles

2 spring onions, shredded

Directions

STEP 1

Heat half the oil in a frying pan over a medium heat. Add the mushrooms and fry for 5-6 mins, or until golden. Transfer to a bowl using a slotted spoon and set aside. Add the remaining oil to the pan and fry the tofu for 3-4 mins, or until evenly golden.

STEP 2

Mix the miso paste with 325ml boiling water in a jug. Cook the noodles following pack instructions, then drain and transfer to a bowl. Top with the mushrooms and tofu, then pour over the miso broth. Scatter over the spring onions just before serving.

Curried kale & chickpea soup

Ingredients

1 tsp rapeseed or coconut oil

1 onion, chopped

1 tbsp grated ginger

2 garlic cloves, crushed

1 sweet potato (about 200g), peeled and cut into 2cm cubes

1 tsp turmeric

2 tsp ground cumin

2 tbsp medium or hot curry powder

400g can chickpeas, rinsed

150ml low-fat coconut milk

500ml vegetable stock (see tip, below)

160g kale, chopped

1 lime, juiced

1 red chilli, finely chopped (optional)

Directions

STEP 1

Heat the oil in a large pan and fry the onion for 5 mins. Add the ginger and garlic, fry for 1 min more, then stir in the sweet potato, spices and chickpeas. Cook for another 5 mins, adding a little water if the spices stick to the pan.

STEP 2

Pour in the coconut milk and 400ml of the stock, then bring to a simmer and cook for 8 mins. Season, then transfer a quarter of the soup to a blender and whizz until smooth. Pour in the reserved stock to loosen, if needed, then add back to the pan with the remaining soup. Stir in the kale and cook for 5 mins. Add the lime juice, then ladle into bowls and scatter over the chilli, if you like.

Butter bean curry wraps

Ingredients

2 large wholemeal tortilla wraps

½ the butter bean curry (recipe below)

2 handfuls of mixed salad leaves

½ the raita (recipe below)

Directions

STEP 1

Warm the wraps following pack instructions, or for
a few seconds on each side over the gas flame of the
hob to create a slight char.

STEP 2

Reheat leftover butter bean curry in a pan over a low
heat until piping hot (if it's quite wet, allow it to
reduce slightly). Spread the curry over the centre of
the wraps, then top with the salad and the raita. Roll
up tightly and serve straightaway.

Baked ginger & spinach sweet potato

Ingredients

1 sweet potato

2 tsp oil

½ onion, finely chopped

1 garlic clove, crushed

small knob of ginger, grated

1-2 tsp curry paste (use what you have or buy a Madras or red curry paste)

knob of butter

handful of spinach

Directions

STEP 1

Heat oven to 200C/180C fan/gas 6. Prick the potato and bake it for 40-45 mins or until soft when you squeeze the sides.

STEP 2

Meanwhile, heat the oil in a small frying pan and fry the onion until softened, add the garlic and cook for 1 min, then add the ginger and curry paste and cook for another min. Stir in the butter and spinach, and continue stirring until the spinach wilts. Season well.

STEP 3

Cut open the top of the sweet potato, scoop out some of the flesh, add it to the mix in the pan and stir through, then spoon the mixture back into the potato.

South Indian coconut & prawn curry

Ingredients

1 large onion, quartered

0.5 thumb-sized piece ginger (no need to peel)

4 garlic cloves

4 tomatoes, 2 halved, 2 cut into wedges

2 tsp rapeseed oil

½ cinnamon stick

½ tsp black mustard seeds

3 cloves

seeds from 4 cardamom pods, crushed

½ tsp ground turmeric

1 tsp ground coriander

10 fresh or dried curry leaves

½ fish stock cube

15g creamed coconut, chopped

1 red chilli, halved, deseeded and sliced or diced

150g pack raw, shelled king prawns

140g skinless cod, cut in half, then halve again to make chunky strips

Directions

STEP 1

Put the onion, ginger, garlic and the halved tomatoes in a food processor with 50ml water and blitz to a smooth purée. You may need to scrape down the inside of the food processor a couple of times. Heat the oil in a large, deep non-stick frying pan, pour in the purée, cover with a lid and cook for 10 mins.

STEP 2

Add the 1/2 cinnamon stick, mustard seeds, cloves, cardamom, turmeric, coriander and curry leaves, and cook for a few mins, stirring. Pour in 300ml water with the stock cube, coconut and chilli, then leave to simmer for 10 mins more. Taste to ensure that the onion is fully cooked – if not, it is worth cooking for another 5 mins.

STEP 3

Finally, add the tomato wedges, prawns and fish, gently stir into the sauce, then cover and cook for 5 mins. Serve with the Spicy cauliflower pilau (see Goes well with).

Black-eyed bean mole with salsa

Ingredients

For the salsa

1 red onion, finely chopped

2 large tomatoes, chopped

2 tbsp fresh coriander

½ lime, zest and juice

For the mole

2 tsp rapeseed oil

1 red onion, halved and sliced

1 garlic clove, finely grated

1 tsp ground coriander

1 tsp mild chilli powder

½ tsp ground cinnamon

400g can black-eyed beans in water

2 tsp cocoa

1 tsp vegetable bouillon

1 tbsp tomato purée

Directions

STEP 1

Tip all the salsa Ingredients into a bowl and stir together.

STEP 2

For the mole, heat the oil in a non-stick pan, add the onion and garlic and fry stirring frequently until softened. Tip in the spices, stir then add the contents of the can of beans with the cocoa, bouillon and tomato purée. Cook, stirring frequently to make quite a thick sauce.

STEP 3

Spoon into shallow bowls, top with the salsa and serve.

Mushroom jacket potatoes

Ingredients

2 large potatoes

2 tsp sunflower oil

250g mushrooms

100g sour cream & chive dip

sprigs of dill (to garnish)

Directions

STEP 1

Heat oven to 200C/180C fan/gas 6. Prick the potatoes all over with a fork and rub with half the sunflower oil. Bake the potatoes for 1 hr 20 mins.

STEP 2

Slice the mushrooms, fry in the remaining oil, then stir through the sour cream & chive dip.

DELIGHTFUL RECIPES FOR DINNER

Sweetcorn & courgette fritters

Ingredients

198g can sweetcorn, drained

2 spring onions, finely chopped

50g courgette, grated

1 tsp smoked paprika

50g self-raising flour

5 eggs, 1 beaten, 4 for poaching

40ml milk

4 tbsp sweet chilli sauce

juice 1 lime

1 tbsp vegetable oil

mixed leaves, to serve

Directions

STEP 1

Mix the sweetcorn, spring onions, courgette, paprika, flour, beaten egg, milk and some seasoning in a large bowl and set aside.

STEP 2

Put a large pan of water on to boil. In a bowl, mix the chilli sauce with the lime juice and set aside.

STEP 3

Heat the oil in a large, non-stick pan and spoon in four burger-sized mounds of the fritter mixture, spaced apart (you may need to do this in two batches). When brown on the underside, turn over and cook for 3 mins more until golden.

STEP 4

Meanwhile, poach the eggs in the simmering water for 2-3 mins until cooked and the yolks are runny. Remove with a slotted spoon. Serve the fritters topped with a poached egg, mixed leaves and a drizzle of the chilli dressing.

Moroccan roast lamb with roasted roots & coriander

Ingredients

½ leg of lamb, around 800g

2 red onions, cut into wedges

1 butternut squash, skin left on, cut into wedges

1 celeriac, peeled and cut into wedges

2½ tbsp cold pressed rapeseed oil

2 tbsp ras el hanout

8 garlic cloves, skin on

1 small bunch coriander

½ tsp cumin seeds

1 lemon, zested and juiced

½ green chilli, deseeded

Directions

STEP 1

Take the lamb out of the fridge while you chop the onions, squash and celeriac. Heat oven to

200C/180C fan/gas 6. Trim any excess fat off the leg of lamb, then cut a few slashes into the meat. Rub ½ tbsp oil and 1 tbsp ras el hanout over the lamb and season with salt and pepper. Put the onion, celeriac, butternut squash into a large roasting tin with the garlic. Toss with the remaining ras el hanout, remaining oil and some salt and pepper. Nestle the lamb into the tin and put in the oven to roast for 40 mins.

STEP 2

Take the lamb out of the oven and leave to rest. Put the veg back in the oven for 20 mins. Meanwhile, blitz the coriander, cumin seeds, lemon zest, lemon juice and green chilli together in a mini food processor until finely chopped and vivid green.

STEP 3

Carve the lamb, put on a platter, then pile on the veg. Sprinkle over some of the coriander mixture before taking the platter to the table for everyone to help themselves.

Easy broccoli pasta

Ingredients

1 head of broccoli, chopped into florets

1 garlic clove, unpeeled

2 tbsp olive oil

250g pasta shells

½ small pack parsley

½ small pack basil

30g toasted pine nuts

½ lemon, zested and juiced

30g parmesan (or vegetarian alternative), plus extra to serve

Directions

STEP 1

Heat the oven to 200C/180C fan/gas 6. Toss the broccoli and garlic in 1 tbsp of the olive oil on a roasting tray and roast in the oven for 10-12 mins, until softened.

STEP 2

Tip the pasta shells into a pan of boiling, salted water. Cook according to packet instructions and drain. Tip the parsley, basil, pine nuts, lemon juice and parmesan into a blender. Once the broccoli is done, set aside a few of the smaller pieces. Squeeze the garlic from its skin, add to the blender along with the rest of the broccoli, pulse to a pesto and season well.

STEP 3

Toss the pasta with the pesto. Add the reserved broccoli florets, split between two bowls and top with a little extra parmesan, the lemon zest and a good grinding of black pepper, if you like.

Salmon salad with sesame dressing

Ingredients

For the salad

250g new potatoes, sliced

160g French beans, trimmed

2 wild salmon fillets

80g salad leaves

4 small clementines, 3 sliced, 1 juiced

handful of basil, chopped

handful of coriander, chopped

For the dressing

2 tsp sesame oil

2 tsp tamari

½ lemon, juiced

1 red chilli, deseeded and chopped

2 tbsp finely chopped onion (¼ small onion)

Directions

STEP 1

Steam the potatoes and beans in a steamer basket set over a pan of boiling water for 8 mins. Arrange the salmon fillets on top and steam for a further 6-8 mins, or until the salmon flakes easily when tested with a fork.

STEP 2

Meanwhile, mix the dressing Ingredients together along with the clementine juice. If eating straightaway, divide the salad leaves between two plates and top with the warm potatoes and beans and the clementine slices. Arrange the salmon fillets on top, scatter over the herbs and spoon over the dressing. If taking to work, prepare the potatoes, beans and salmon the night before, then pack into a rigid airtight container with the salad leaves kept separate. Put the salad elements together and dress just before eating to prevent the leaves from wilting.

Pot-roast beef with French onion gravy

Ingredients

1kg silverside or topside of beef with no added fat

2 tbsp olive oil

8 young carrots, tops trimmed (but leave a little, if
you like)

1 celery stick, finely chopped

200ml white wine

600ml rich beef stock

2 bay leaves

500g onion

a few thyme sprigs

1 tsp butter

1 tsp light brown or light muscovado sugar

2 tsp plain flour

Directions

STEP 1

Heat oven to 160C/140C fan/gas 3. Rub the meat with 1 tsp of the oil and plenty of seasoning. Heat a large flameproof casserole dish and brown the meat all over for about 10 mins. Meanwhile, add 2 tsp oil to a frying pan and fry the carrots and celery for 10 mins until turning golden.

STEP 2

Lift the beef onto a plate, splash the wine into the hot casserole and boil for 2 mins. Pour in the stock, return the beef, then tuck in the carrots, celery and bay leaves, trying not to submerge the carrots too much. Cover and cook in the oven for 2 hrs. (I like to turn the beef halfway through cooking.)

STEP 3

Meanwhile, thinly slice the onions. Heat 1 tbsp oil in a pan and stir in the onions, thyme and some seasoning. Cover and cook gently for 20 mins until the onions are softened but not coloured. Remove the lid, turn up the heat, add the butter and sugar, then let the onions caramelise to a dark golden brown, stirring often. Remove the thyme sprigs, then set aside.

STEP 4

When the beef is ready, it will be tender and easy to pull apart at the edges. Remove it from the casserole and snip off the strings. Reheat the onion pan, stir in the flour and cook for 1 min. Whisk the floury onions into the beefy juices in the casserole, to make a thick onion gravy. Taste for seasoning. Add the beef and carrots back to the casserole, or slice the beef and bring to the table on a platter, with the carrots to the side and the gravy spooned over.

Roasted aloo gobi

Ingredients

400g floury potatoes (such as Maris Piper or King Edward), cut into medium-sized chunks

1 large cauliflower, cut into florets

1 tbsp cumin seeds

2 tsp coriander seeds

2 tsp nigella seeds

1 tsp ground cinnamon

1 tsp turmeric

1 tsp chilli powder

4 tbsp vegetable oil or sunflower oil or rapeseed oil

8 curry leaves

4 garlic cloves, crushed

2 x 400g cans chopped tomatoes

2 small green chillies, pierced a few times

1 tsp golden caster sugar

1 lime, juiced

small pack coriander, chopped

basmati rice, naan and natural yogurt, to serve

Directions

STEP 1

Heat oven to 180C/160C fan/gas 4. Tip the potatoes into a large pan, fill with cold water and bring to the boil. Simmer for 5-6 mins until starting to soften but still holding their shape. Drain well.

STEP 2

On a large baking tray, toss the potatoes and cauliflower with the spices and 2 tbsp oil. Season well and roast for 45 mins, stirring halfway through cooking, until the veg is soft and starting to brown.

STEP 3

Meanwhile, heat the remaining oil in a large pan. Fry the curry leaves and garlic for 1 min, making sure the garlic doesn't brown. Add the tomatoes, chillies, sugar, lime juice and some seasoning.

Cover with a lid and simmer for 15 mins until the tomatoes have broken down.

STEP 4

Add the roasted veg to the tomatoes. Simmer for 5 mins, adding a splash of water if the curry gets too thick. Stir through the coriander and serve with rice, warm naan and yogurt.

Pepper & lemon spaghetti with basil & pine nuts

Ingredients

1 tbsp rapeseed oil

1 red pepper, deseeded and diced

150g wholemeal spaghetti

2 courgettes (250g), grated

2 garlic cloves, finely grated

1 lemon, zested and juiced

15g basil, finely chopped

25g pine nuts, toasted

2 tbsp finely grated parmesan or vegetarian alternative (optional)

Directions

STEP 1

Heat the oil in a large non-stick frying pan. Add the pepper and cook for 5 mins. Meanwhile, cook the pasta for 10-12 mins until tender.

STEP 2

Add the courgette and garlic to the pepper and cook, stirring very frequently, for 10-15 mins until the courgette is really soft.

STEP 3

Stir in the lemon zest and juice, basil and spaghetti (reserve some pasta water) and toss together, adding a little of the pasta water until nicely coated. Add the pine nuts, then spoon into bowls and serve topped with the parmesan, if using.

DELIGHTFUL RECIPES FOR DESSERT

Frozen yogurt

Ingredients

200g strawberries,

300g Greek or Greek-style yogurt

4 tbsp condensed milk

Directions

STEP 1

Use a food processor or blender to blitz the strawberries for a smoother end result, or crush them in a bowl using a fork to get chunkier pieces.

STEP 2

Tip the yogurt and condensed milk into the food processor or blender with the strawberries and blitz again to combine.

STEP 3

Pour into a freezer-proof container and put in the freezer, stirring every hour to break up the ice crystals, then leave to freeze again overnight. Remove from the freezer 10 mins before serving.

Vegan brownies

Ingredients

2 tbsp ground flaxseed

200g dark chocolate, roughly chopped

½ tsp coffee granules

80g vegan margarine, plus extra for greasing

125g self-raising flour

70g ground almonds

50g cocoa powder

¼ tsp baking powder

250g golden caster sugar

1½ tsp vanilla extract

Directions

STEP 1

Heat the oven to 170C/150C fan/gas 3½. Grease and line a 20cm square tin with baking parchment. Combine the flaxseed with 6 tbsp water and set aside for at least 5 mins.

STEP 2

In a saucepan, melt 120g chocolate, the coffee and margarine with 60ml water on a low heat. Allow to cool slightly.

STEP 3

Put the flour, almonds, cocoa, baking powder and ¼ tsp salt in a bowl and stir to remove any lumps. Using a hand whisk, mix the sugar into the melted chocolate mixture, and beat well until smooth and glossy, ensuring all the sugar is well dissolved. Stir in the flaxseed mixture, vanilla extract and remaining chocolate, then the flour mixture. Spoon into the prepared tin.

STEP 4

Bake for 35-45 mins until a skewer inserted in the middle comes out clean with moist crumbs. Allow to cool in the tin completely, then cut into squares. Store in an airtight container and eat within three days.

Healthy banana bread

Ingredients

low-fat spread, for the tin, plus extra to serve

140g wholemeal flour

100g self-raising flour

1 tsp bicarbonate of soda

1 tsp baking powder

300g mashed banana from overripe black bananas

4 tbsp agave syrup

3 large eggs, beaten with a fork

150ml pot low-fat natural yogurt

25g chopped pecan or walnuts (optional)

Directions

STEP 1

Heat oven to 160C/140C fan/gas 3. Grease and line a
2lb loaf tin with baking parchment (allow it to come
2cm above top of tin). Mix the flours, bicarb, baking
powder and a pinch of salt in a large bowl.

STEP 2

Mix the bananas, syrup, eggs and yogurt. Quickly
stir into dry Ingredients, then gently scrape into the

tin and scatter with nuts, if using. Bake for 1 hr 10 mins-1 hr 15 mins or until a skewer comes out clean.

STEP 3

Cool in tin on a wire rack. Eat warm or at room temperature, with low-fat spread.

Avocado & strawberry ices

Ingredients

200g ripe strawberries, hulled and chopped

1 avocado, stoned, peeled and roughly chopped

2 tsp balsamic vinegar

½ tsp vanilla extract

1-2 tsp maple syrup (optional)

Directions

STEP 1

Put the strawberries (save four pieces for the top), avocado, vinegar and vanilla in a bowl and blitz using a hand blender (or in a food processor) until as smooth as you can get it. Have a taste and only add the maple syrup if the strawberries are not sweet enough.

STEP 2

Pour into containers, add a strawberry to each, cover with cling film and freeze. Allow the pots to soften for 5-10 mins before eating.

Easy crêpes

Ingredients

175g plain flour

3 large eggs

450ml milk

sunflower oil, for frying

Directions

STEP 1

Weigh the flour in a large jug or bowl. Crack in the eggs, add half the milk and a pinch of salt. Whisk to a smooth, thick batter. Add the remaining milk and whisk again. Set aside for at least 30 mins.

STEP 2

Heat a large non-stick crêpe pan or frying pan. Add a drizzle of oil, then wipe out the excess with kitchen paper. When the pan is hot, add enough batter to just cover the surface, swirling it and pouring any excess back into the bowl. The pancake should be as thin as possible. When the edges are peeling away from the sides of the pan, shake it to see if the pancake easily releases and is browning on the underside. If not, cook a little longer. Flip and cook the other side for a minute or two. Serve, or keep warm in a low oven.

Sugar-free banana bread

Ingredients

125g self-raising wholemeal flour

½ tsp baking powder

2 tsp ground cinnamon

75g sultana

50g butter, melted

2 tsp vanilla essence

1 egg

1 tbsp milk

3 ripe bananas, mashed

drizzle agave syrup, to serve (optional)

Directions

STEP 1

Grown ups: Preheat the oven to 180C/ 160C fan/ gas mark 4. Grease and line a 450g loaf/1lb tin with baking parchment.

STEP 2

Children: Weigh the flour, baking powder, cinnamon and sultanas into a bowl and mix with a wooden spoon. Then weigh the butter, vanilla essence, egg, milk and mashed bananas and put into another bowl or jug and mix with a small balloon whisk or fork. Pour the 'wet' banana mixture into the 'dry' flour mixture and combine thoroughly with a wooden spoon. Weighing needs to be very accurate when baking so help older children to measure carefully. Younger children can also get involved by spooning or pouring into the scales with adult supervision. Younger children can also beat the egg with a fork and mash the banana with a potato masher.

STEP 3

Grown ups: Pour the cake mixture into the prepared tin and bake for 30 - 40 mins or until a skewer inserted in the middle comes out clean. Remove from the oven, allow to cool in the tin for 10 mins then turn out.

STEP 4

Children: Drizzle with agave syrup if using.

Vegan banana pancakes

Ingredients

1 large ripe banana (around 150g)

2 tbsp golden caster sugar

¼ tsp fine salt

2 tbsp vegetable oil, plus extra for cooking

120g self-raising flour

½ tsp baking powder

150ml oat, almond milk or soya milk

syrup, sliced banana and berries, to serve (optional)

Directions

STEP 1

Mash the banana in a mixing bowl. Stir in the sugar, salt and oil. Add the flour and baking powder and mix thoroughly. Make a well in the centre and gradually whisk in the milk. The batter should be a thick, droppable consistency.

STEP 2

Heat a little oil in a frying pan over a medium heat. Add 2 tbsp of the batter to make American-style pancakes. You will be able to make about 4-5 at a time. Fry on each side for 2-3 mins until golden. Serve with syrup, sliced banana and berries, if you like.

8

TO WRAP THINGS UP!

To successfully adopt and maintain a high protein, high fiber, low-calorie lifestyle, it's essential to make thoughtful choices in both your diet and daily habits. This approach revolves around prioritizing nutrient-dense foods that provide ample protein and fiber while keeping calorie intake moderate.

Begin by understanding the core principles of this lifestyle. High protein sources include lean meats like chicken and turkey, fish, eggs, dairy products such as Greek yogurt, and plant-based options like beans and tofu. For fiber, focus on incorporating fruits such as berries and apples, vegetables like leafy greens and broccoli, whole grains such as oats and quinoa, as well as nuts, seeds, and legumes.

Effective meal planning is crucial. Aim to balance your macronutrients in each meal, ensuring a mix of protein, fiber, and healthy fats. Meal prepping can help you avoid unhealthy food choices by having nutritious meals ready ahead of time and practicing portion control.

When choosing foods, opt for lean proteins such as skinless poultry and fish, whole grains over refined grains, and a variety of colorful fruits and vegetables. Hydration is also key; drink plenty of water throughout the day to support digestion and maintain satiety.

Incorporating regular physical activity is recommended to complement dietary changes, promoting metabolism and preserving muscle mass. Adequate sleep is equally important for overall health and appetite regulation, aiming for 7-9 hours per night.

To avoid common pitfalls, limit processed foods high in sugars and unhealthy fats, as well as alcoholic beverages and sugary drinks. Keeping a food journal can help track your progress and identify areas for improvement, alongside monitoring weight loss and body measurements.

Finding support can enhance your journey. Consider joining online communities or local groups focused on healthy eating for motivation and advice. Seeking guidance from a dietitian or nutritionist can provide personalized strategies for long-term success.

Lastly, maintain flexibility in your approach. Incorporate mindful eating practices to enjoy your meals fully and recognize when you're satisfied. Including occasional treats can prevent feelings of deprivation and help sustain your commitment over time.

By integrating these strategies consistently into your lifestyle, you can establish and sustain a high protein, high fiber, low-calorie way of eating that promotes overall health and well-being effectively.